The Drink Beer, Get Thin Diet

A Low Carbohydrate Approach

By

Bob Skilnik

ISBN: 1-4107-3386-6 (e-book)
ISBN: 1-4107-3385-8 (Paperback)

This book is printed on acid free paper.

1stBooks – rev. 04/28/03

Acknowledgements

Information on the carbohydrate content of more than 350 brands of beers listed in the book was graciously provided by over fifty worldwide breweries. Their help and cooperation is what made this book possible and allowed me to shed over fifty-five pounds and five pant sizes.

Last, but not least, thanks to my wife, Daria, who stills thinks a tried and true beer diet is a crazy concept but can now get her hands around my waist.

Contents

Preface

An Overview

That's Not A Beer-Belly

If the "six-pack abs" of your youth now look more like a half-barrel of beer hanging over your belly, **The Drink Beer, Get Thin Diet** is for you. If you're a chronic dieter who wants (and needs) results but won't give up the occasional libation, here's the diet you've been looking for! With careful monitoring of your daily carbohydrate intake, you'll be able to enjoy two or more beers a day and still lose weight.

But beer, some skeptical readers might ask? Isn't beer fattening? Isn't beer the reason you're lugging around that beer-belly today? Not necessarily, but if you're slamming down a six-pack or two a week of your favorite brew, accompanied with pizza specials, cheeseburgers on onion rolls with all the toppings, chips and dip and unlimited amounts of other carbohydrate-laden snacks, well then yes, beer might be a small part of your weight problem, a very small part.

For most of us chronic dieters who have spent our early years gorging on food and drink, the consistent practices of poor eating and drinking habits, a slower metabolism and the ravages of Father Time have led us down the inevitable path of obesity.

This kind of Falstaffian eating and drinking practice brings up a word I'm sure you've heard before, the word that really is the key to this or any weight reduction program—*moderation*. This means eating sufficient amounts of body-building protein, generous portions of green vegetables and fresh fruit, some necessary fat and a balanced amount of carbohydrates. It also means one or two 12-ounce bottles or cans of beer a day, possibly three servings during the weekends.

A Beer Diet? Why Not?

Beer in moderation has long been advocated by the United States brewing industry as a healthful temperance drink, a *"...drink of moderation."* Before National Prohibition, the industry habitually claimed all kinds of healthful benefits from beer, some claims bordering on the ludicrous. When beer was again legalized in 1933, advertisements listing the nutritional content of beer were often touted by the brewing industry.

Government food and nutritional regulations, however, no longer permit health claims for beer. But in our enlightened present era, the United States Agriculture Department, in conjunction with the Department of Health and Human Services, recently allowed as to how moderate drinking may actually be beneficial to folks. Their studies concluded that fourteen 12-ounce bottles of beer a week are an acceptable part of a normal balanced diet, half that if you're a woman. Maybe the old time brewers with their advertising hyperbole actually knew what they were talking about!

Our English friends take the recommendation for a healthy weekly beer allowance even further. The British government recently sanctioned the consumption of up to 18 bottles of beer or ale a week for men and 14 bottles for women, as part of an acceptable diet. The Germans, acknowledged connoisseurs of beer-making and drinking, have not only observed that the moderate consumption of beer can be a healthy part of a daily diet, they recently concluded that small amounts of beer might even retard aging.

Okay. With those few paragraphs, maybe I've convinced a few of you that a moderate amount of beer can be a healthful part of your diet. Some of you, I know, are probably an easy sell when it comes to claims of beer as a healthful and stimulating tonic; but what about the doubting Thomas' out there? Still not sure that beer in moderate amounts can not only be good for you but can also be a part of a weight reduction program? To carry the argument a step further, several of you might even be asking how a regular beer drinking kind of guy gets off writing this book, playing the part of a diet expert? Well, to paraphrase a too often clichéd television commercial, *"I'm not a Doctor. I don't even play one on TV."* I'm just a guy who has tried every diet that's come out in the last thirty years. I've followed the adventures of *Dr. Atkins' Diet Revolution, Dr. Atkins' New Diet Cookbook, Dr. Stillman's Quick Weight Loss Diet, Dr. Tarnower's Complete Scarsdale Medical Diet, The*

Grapefruit Diet, Protein Power, *The Zone,* and for those of you who couldn't understand the complications of *The Zone...Mastering The Zone,* even the old liquid *Opti-Fast* protein diet, a diet approach that was openly advocated by Oprah Winfrey. Remember Oprah coming on stage at Harpo Studios all slim and trim, dragging a wagon full of yellowed beef fat and tallow behind her, symbolizing the unsightly weight she had lost?

Been there, done that. In fact, I'd venture to say that I've also lost and regained over 800 pounds in the last thirty years, and if I'm correct, I suspect a lot of you have done the same thing. Hit or miss dieting can be torture. During this time, I've starved and tormented myself through the vast *waist* land of scores of diets and can recite the philosophy of all of them by chapter and verse.

I'm also a dedicated beer drinker. I've enjoyed beers from micros to macros, Old World brew to my own home brew. My knowledge and appreciation of beer were finely honed at the famous Siebel Institute of Technology in Chicago where I studied beer and brewing technology with brewers from Miller, Stroh, Coors, numerous stateside brewpubs, microbreweries and breweries from around the world. I've also tasted a diversity of beers during a three-year stint as a translator in Germany, courtesy of Uncle Sam. I know beer.

When I'm not writing about, making or drinking beer, I've also found time to be a recreational cook. I like to surprise my family and friends with new food recipes and old favorites. Years ago, I owned a small delicatessen in Chicago where I got a feel for enjoyable, good tasting food, especially soups and salads, and the staple of any good deli, the nosh platter. I know food.

But it was this combination of overly enjoying both food and beer, mixed with my own pathetic hulking mass of 305 pounds on a six foot, two inch frame that made me research the sort of diet that would allow me to still enjoy my beer and even snack when hungry.

My best weight loss results have always been achieved with low carbohydrate dieting. I noticed, however, that those low carb diet plans that allowed some beer in their weight loss approach always fixated on low carbohydrate brews. At first, this seemed like an easy approach to low carb dieting. After all, if the logic behind low carb dieting is to restrict foods like potatoes, rice, and bread, it does make sense to drink light beer. However, as you approach your target weight, every low carb diet will allow you to gradually increase your daily carbohydrate intake. That potato you once craved…finally, have one. One, mind you, but moderation, after all, is the key to any weight maintenance program. Have that rice. Have that pasta. Have it all, in moderation, of course, but there's no mention whatsoever about eventually increasing your beer intake to include regular-brewed beers. The observation I had seemed to find a bump, or perhaps a dead-end, in the logic of the most popular low carb diets. If one can increase the carbohydrate level of food…why not the carbohydrate level of beer? Is one to believe that the successful dieter, initially using a low carbohydrate diet would have to spend the rest of his or her life drinking light beer? I don't think so, but every popular low carb diet out there fails to address this issue. Part of this problem has to do with the simple fact that the carbohydrate contents of regular-brewed beers are not emblazoned on their labels or cans. The extensive list of the carbohydrate contents of both light and regular-brewed beers in Chapter 6 takes care of this problem.

The acts of dieting and drinking beer are thought of as two mutually exclusive events. But with all my diet experience, an extensive knowledge of beer and a love of good tasting food, all steeped in a bit of self-experimentation, I now know that a weight reduction regime consisting of a satisfying level of body-building protein, green vegetables, balanced amounts of carbohydrates and a moderate amount of tasty beer can help control my weight. By documenting my success in achieving a significant weight loss with a balance of good nutrition, great recipes, moderate exercise and a wide diversity of beers, I'm sure I can convince you that this enjoyable and effective approach to weight loss will also work for you.

Some Many Beers, So Little Time

The beer revolution of the last decade makes it exceedingly easy to follow **The Drink Beer, Get Thin Diet**. With the staggering selection of beers that now confronts the average beer drinker, your choices of brew are virtually unlimited on this proven diet. Many of the world's leading breweries have graciously provided carbohydrate information of their products for use in this diet. I have included an extensive listing of over 350 brands from more than fifty worldwide breweries to help you control your total daily carbohydrate intake, the key to success in this diet. Hoppy pale ales, golden-colored pilsners, spicy wheat beers, rich and creamy stouts, fruit-flavored beers, tart Belgian chimays…the list of today's beer styles goes on and on.

Even the slumbering national brands have taken notice of this beer revolution. Many of them are now offering their own interpretations of these long-forgotten styles of beer, all making **The Drink Beer, Get Thin Diet** an exciting dietary breakthrough for anyone who wants to lose weight and still enjoy their beer. This diet truly takes the approach of *"having your cake and eating it too."* In this case, however, it's beer we're talking about!

My approach however, is not meant to replace your doctor's advice. If you are diabetic or taking medication, suspect you are sick or are just unsure as to how this diet of moderation might affect you, I insist you see your physician before starting out on this dieting adventure. If you eat out during this weight reduction program and imbibe, recognize the potential dangers of drinking and driving. Finally, if you are a chronic abuser of alcohol, this diet is not for you. Please see your doctor for advice and counseling.

Recipes? Of Course

To further the idea that beer can be a tasteful component of a healthy lifestyle and an easy-to-follow weight loss program, I have included a selection of low carbohydrate recipes that occasionally include beer as a flavorful ingredient. It's certainly not necessary to use these recipes as a component of **The Drink Beer, Get Thin Diet**, however. As long as you keep within the limits of daily carbohydrate consumption, any entrée, soup or salad will do just fine.

Some of the dishes I've included might even require more time than you want to spend in the kitchen during the busy working week. I understand. With a working-professional wife, two hyperactive teenage boys, two goofy dogs (or is that the other way around?) and an eighty-mile round trip commute for my wife and me, it can get pretty hectic around our household from Monday through Friday.

No problem. There are also quick and simple dishes included in the recipe section, taking your busy weekday schedule into account.

Keeping Busy During the Diet

It's on the less hectic weekends when I often use my culinary skills and so should you. During the development and testing of the recipes in this book, I found that weekend cooking helped keep me from faltering. An idle mind is a devil's workshop, and when you're dieting, he seems to work overtime on Saturdays and Sundays. With my own limitations in mind, I would suggest to aspiring dieters that the weekend be used as a great time to not only prepare dishes for the evening, but to also keep yourself busy crafting satisfying and tasteful dishes that can be enjoyed throughout the week. From Monday through Friday, just pull your pre-measured portion from the freezer, nuke it or warm it up on the stove and enjoy it with your evening beer.

What if you don't cook? Why not learn? Not only will cooking keep you pleasantly busy and broaden your gustatory horizons, it just might even give you a little bit of "in" with your wife or girlfriend. *"You relax today honey. I'm marinating chicken fajitas for the grill. By the way, there's a warm Brie with peach preserves in the oven and some cold Coronas in the fridge. I'll have it all ready in a few minutes."* Suddenly you're more than an ordinary beer-drinking kind of guy; you're a compassionate man of the new millennium.

Weekends, Parties, Beer and the Diet

This diet approach openly welcomes weekends, often considered the dark hole of all diets. It's the time of the week when most dieters fail. *"I'll start again on Monday,"* is the customary excuse. I'm sure you know what I'm talking about. On a traditional low calorie diet, there you are, watching a great weekend football game with a boring salad and a big glass of diet soda in front of you. Before the first quarter has ended, you're off your diet. I don't blame you. Most low calorie diets are dull, uninspiring and unforgiving.

How about those dreaded weekend parties? It's certainly no fun to stand in the corner sipping on a glass of seltzer water with a twist of lemon and watching everybody else belly up to the dips and snacks, beer in hand. In my pre-**Drink Beer, Grow Thin Diet** days, whenever I had tried to shed a few pounds, I would often turn into a hermit, unnecessarily avoiding parties whenever possible until I got back down to my target weight.

On **The Drink Beer, Get Thin Diet** with its generous allowance of beer and snacks, you can remain the social butterfly that you always were and still lose weight.

Weekends are also the time when you actually get to "cheat". Want a couple of pieces of salami with your beer? Maybe throw in some crackers? A handful of peanuts? Heck, how about a delicious antipasto plate? Buffalo wings? Maybe you like creamy dips? Why not enjoy a clam dip or onion dip, even a spicy salsa? It's O.K. on this diet. Why not wash it all down with a couple of beers? That's not dieting…that's living!

So, let's get started. Years ago, when I had enlisted in the Army, my father gave me some final words of advice as I left for boot camp, *"Son, I'm telling you, never volunteer for anything!"* However, if I'm to convince you that this diet is real, that it worked for me and can work for you, I'm volunteering to share my dieting experiences with you.

You've got nothing to lose except that "beer-belly."

Chapter 1

Beer Is For Losers

Beer & Food

On April 7, 1933, twenty-three states threw off the first layer of the Volstead Act and resumed the legal brewing of beer with an alcoholic content of 3.2% alcohol by weight. Brewers quickly adapted to their new circumstances and recognized the wisdom of marketing beer as a food product. For the first time ever, packaged beer and food were sold under the same roof, a staple of the present day "Supermarket" concept. Mom could now pick up a week's worth of groceries for the family and a case of beer for Dad (and maybe Mom, too!) in one convenient stop.

In the seventy years or so since beer began sharing grocery shelves with food, we've learned to associate beer drinking with the eating of certain types of food. Beer goes with pizza, reuben sandwiches, steak, ribs, ethnic foods (the spicier, the better), pretzels, peanuts, pop corn, potato chips…the list goes on and on.

Now be honest. When's the last time you enjoyed one single piece of pizza, washed down with only one can of beer? With our combined gorging of food and beer, we've mistakenly begun to think of beer as fattening; it's really not. Most beers average only around 160 calories and 12 grams of carbohydrates per 12-ounce serving, less than a can of regular Coke. But whereas you wouldn't conceive of downing a six-pack of soda in one sitting, pounding back a "sixer" of your favorite malted beverage can be a common occurrence, with you eventually consuming around 1000 calories and over 70 grams of carbohydrates in the process. After about three or four tasty libations, your inhibitions often ease up and the food cravings really begin. Suddenly, one piece of pizza just won't do the trick; two, three, four or five pieces seem about right. The same goes for finger foods and snacks. One handful can inevitably lead to another.

Your Day of Reckoning

Twenty or thirty years of this behavior can take its toll on that once rock-hard body that served you well all those years. But one day, you're looking in the closet for a loose-fitting pair of pants when you discover a dozen pair hanging in the back of the closet that no longer fit you. You don't throw them out, however, insisting that one day you'll lose some weight and wear them again. It's not until you realize that most of those pants are twenty-five year old polyesters that you know you've got a problem. Maybe there's been a time in the last few years when you sheepishly looked in the mirror after stepping out of the shower and tried sucking in your belly. *"My God,"* you say to yourself, *"I'm getting a beer-belly!"*

You start to grunt when you bend over to tie your shoes, but it can get worse. You might fool yourself a little bit longer about your excess baggage, but what about the recent comments from your mate? Has she started to kid you about your *"love handles?"* Has she starting calling you *"Big Guy,"* but for all the wrong reasons? Her remarks might not initially bother you but why let her little "jokes" go any further?

Has the excess weight slowed down or limited your...(*ahem*) sexual performance? A recent study from the Harvard School of Public Health suggests the size of a man's waist might have a relationship with a man's ability to have an erection. Men with a 42-inch waist were nearly twice as likely than men with a 32-inch waist to report *"poor"* or *"very poor"* ability to achieve an erection in a four-week period. This was after accounting for age, smoking and hypertension, all risk factors for impotence. Sure, you're not a young buck anymore. The hairline's receding and you're already using Rogaine but do you really want to add Viagra to your shopping list?

Calorie-wise, carbohydrate-wise, fat-wise, it wasn't the beer that single handedly did you in; it was the excessive amounts of high-carbohydrate foods washed down with copious quantities of beer that put those excess pounds on you; a weighty combination.

There is, however, hope for us older studs who have lost weight and have also learned the benefits of moderation in our beer drinking. A Czech doctor says that by drinking beer every day men may keep their sex lives active. *"If men drink two beers a day they can stave off impotence,"* says Dr. Pavel Zemek of the Czech Center of Gerontology in Prague. Zemek says his research shows beer can have a *"powerful effect"* in stopping the arteries from becoming blocked.

"On the basis of clinical tests, we can say moderate amounts of beer lessens arterial sclerosis,

one of the causes of erectile dysfunction," he told a local newspaper.

Beer…The Drink of Moderation

If you want to lose weight on **The Drink Beer, Get Thin Diet**, and you certainly will if you follow this revolutionary plan, you'll need to reevaluate your idea of beer and food. Begin with this simple premise; *beer is a healthy beverage of moderation and can be a pleasant diversion in any balanced adult diet.*

In moderate amounts, beer stimulates appetite and enhances digestion. It is composed mostly of water plus alcohol and some organic and inorganic compounds. Vitamins and minerals in beer include potassium, calcium, niacin, vitamins B1, B2 and B6. When consumed in moderate amounts and combined with a diet of protein, vegetables, fruit and some carbohydrates, the alcoholic properties of beer can promote a relaxed and therapeutic effect on the adult individual.

Even the U.S. Government has recognized the benefits of moderate beer consumption. Philip R. Lee, former Assistant Secretary of U.S. Health and Human Services, commenting after the release of a government study titled the <u>Dietary Guidelines for Americans</u>, pointed out that drinking *"…in moderation, with meals and when consumption does not put you or others at risk…can be…fine for health."* The government report, issued jointly with the Agriculture Department, is a compilation of foods and eating habits advocated by U.S. experts for good health. It's interesting to note that a 1990 statement that *"...drinking has no net health benefit"* was removed from the new report. The study also confirmed something that most of us have known all along. *"Alcoholic beverages have been used to enhance the enjoyment of meals by many societies throughout hum*an *history."*

Finally, your taxpayer's money put to good use!

Added Benefits of Moderate Beer Drinking

Beer does more than add nutritive value to our meals as these findings from numerous beer-oriented web sites point out;

- A Japanese research group has learned that beer may inhibit cancer-causing carcinogens found in charred meats and fish. Something to think about when you're enjoying a beer at your next BBQ.
- British Secretary of State for Health Stephen Dorrell announced, after a government study in which his agency took testimony from nearly 100 organizations, including the British Medical Association and the American Medical Association, that they found that a glass of beer or wine a day is good for men older than 40 and for post-menopausal women.
- Researchers at Indiana University Medical Center, Indianapolis, unexpectedly discovered that moderate drinking not only did no harm, but that the alcohol seemed to improve the

subjects' memories and their problem-solving and reasoning abilities. Those test subjects who reported having one to two drinks a day scored significantly higher on mental skills tests than those who drank either more or less.

- Alcohol appears to protect the heart by raising levels of HDL, the good variety of cholesterol, and it may have other beneficial effects on the circulatory system as well. According to a study reported at the American Heart Association's 70th Scientific Sessions in Orlando, Florida in 1997, the longevity of 4,797 male physicians who had suffered a previous heart attack and 953 who had experienced a stroke, was lengthened for those who consumed up to two alcoholic drinks a day, reducing their chances of premature death and heart attack by 20 to 30 percent. *"We found a clear reduction in the risk of death in light to moderate drinkers compared to people who didn't drink at all,"* reported J. Michael Gaziano, M.D., former director of cardiovascular epidemiology at Boston's Brigham and Women's Hospital, who led the study.

- The question of what is moderate drinking took on a new dimension with a study of heart patients at the Desert Cardiology of Tucson. As Dr. Tedd Goldfinger, senior cardiologist and president of the center noted, *"The fact is, we found that the more you drink, the better the outcome with heart disease—up to a point. But we may not want to present that to the public, because it is probably much more than the public is ready for."* Are you ready?

- A recent study suggests a possible link of alcohol consumption with leanness. Some experts believe that much of the energy in alcohol is quickly burned off as heat and therefore not stored by the body as fat.

- Beer may retard bodily aging. According to a recent European survey, 81% of German general practitioners are convinced that one or two liters (about 33 ounces per liter) of beer daily make life more enjoyable and healthier for the elderly, and as a result, retard aging. You've got to hand it to the Germans. After two quarts of beer, I have to admit that I sometimes feel like I'm a kid again, too.

- A report in an issue of <u>Diabetes</u> also has indicated that drinking on at least 5 days of the week provided the best insurance against developing diabetes, even when the amount of alcohol consumed was minimal. Researchers found that men who consumed 15 to 29 grams of alcohol daily had a 36% lower risk of diabetes over 12 years, compared with men who did not drink and with men who were lighter drinkers.

- A study of over 85,000 women has reported that the heart protecting benefits of alcohol may also apply to women. This study, published in May of 1997 in the <u>New England Journal of Medicine</u>, found that the overall risk of heart attacks among light-to-moderate drinking women was almost 14% lower than the risk for non-drinkers and heavy drinkers. Moreover, there was no evidence that light drinking increased a woman's risk of dying of cancer, a prior concern.

- Michael J. Thun, M.D., of the American Cancer Society in Atlanta has found that *"The cardiovascular benefits of moderate drinking increases with age and in patients with higher cardiovascular-disease risk."*

And finally, this little exchange between Dr. Renaud, a researcher of the so-called "French Paradox," consisting of a diet of high-fat and moderate alcohol consumption and Morley Safer of 60 Minutes:

Dr. RENAUD: *"It's well-documented that really, an intake, a moderate intake of alcohol, prevents coronary heart disease by as much as fifty percent. I mean, this is—"*

SAFER: *"Fifty percent?"*

Dr. RENAUD: *"...fifty percent. I mean, there is no other drug that is being so efficient as a moderate intake of alcohol. Of course, the problem is that people are tempted to go beyond this moderate intake."*

The truth is out there, but as the good doctor points out, moderation is the key to success.

Chapter 2

Carbohydrates and Insulin

Calories Don't Count

No one likes confusing mumbo-jumbo more than me. Therefore, I'll skip as much of the technical information as possible as to why this diet works and get right to the point.

The Drink Beer, Get Thin Diet is based on the theory of lower carbohydrate consumption. Carbohydrates are metabolized as sugar. You probably remember from your high school science class how it's necessary for your body to convert starch (carbohydrates) into sugar (mostly glucose) before it's released into the bloodstream for energy. With a daily intake of about 2,200 calories, assuming a sixty-percent intake of carbohydrates, your body would have to contend with the metabolic equivalent of around two cups of sugar! On most caloric diets, you scrupulously avoid sugar but think nothing of eating starches such as pasta or rice because you've been told how good carbohydrates are for you.

Get the notion out of your head that a low-fat, high carbohydrate diet will lead to a successful reduction in weight. Look at the shelves of your local supermarket; fat free and low fat items are displayed everywhere. This low fat/fat free mania has been going on for years, and yet, we keep reading how the population, as a whole, is overweight and getting heavier. There seems to be a relationship between the onset of the low fat craze in foods, beginning in the 1980s, and the current epidemic of obesity. You've probably been practicing this sort of diet philosophy for years. If you have, put this book down and go look in the mirror. Something wrong with what you see?

That "something" is the result of excessive insulin production. By eating high amounts of carbohydrates, our blood glucose levels rise, forcing a high level of insulin to be released into the bloodstream in order to lower the resultant spike in our blood glucose levels. The insulin converts a portion of the glucose to glycogen, stored in the muscles and liver and readily available for energy use. If all the glycogen storage areas are full, however, insulin will convert the excess glucose into triglycerides, which we carry around on our bodies as adipose tissue, otherwise known as FAT. This rush of insulin also causes an eventual lowering of your blood sugar causing your body to mistakenly think it has run out of fuel. The result? You crave more carbohydrates…and the cycle of eating using carbohydrates for more fuel begins again.

That's as technical as we need to be. In order to lose weight, you must initially restrict foods that stimulate an excessive amount of insulin, i.e., carbohydrates, especially refined carbohydrates.

Now the good part. If a person follows this tenant of simplicity, at almost any level of caloric intake, he or she will lose weight. In other words, calories don't count; carbohydrates do!

However, before we begin, I want to once again reemphasize the absolute importance of checking

with your doctor before beginning any program of weight reduction. A complete battery of blood work tests should be part of your doctor's pre-diet evaluation. The pre-diet blood tests will also give you a base for later comparisons of your progress when you revisit your physician on a regular basis during this weight loss program.

Chapter 3

Light Beer versus Regular Beer

Not Your Father's Beer

If you're assuming that this diet advocates the free wheeling beer consumption that probably got you into a pants size that closely matches your age, you're holding the wrong book in your hands. Your daily allowance of beer will be restricted to no more than 30% of your daily carbohydrate intake. This restriction leaves you with what might initially appear to be a small range of beer choices. This is a common complaint when some dedicated beer drinkers begin **The Drink Beer, Get Thin Diet**. To this, I always like to point out the obvious. *"Show me any other successful and satisfying weight reduction program that allows **any** beer during the diet!"* The full spectrum of low carbohydrate beers on the market today, as well as a smaller selection of regular beers, will help you get through the 30-day Initial Phase of the diet.

There is a small but vocal beer-drinking minority, however, that looks at the manufacture of light beer as an abomination foisted upon the American public by national breweries. A friend who successfully followed the diet bemoaned his limited choices of beer during the Initial Phase. After trying a number of different beers during the first month of **The Drink Beer, Get Thin Diet**, both low carbohydrate and regular-brewed beers, he now enjoys Amstel Light as his beer of choice. He wound up joining the huge segment of beer drinkers that appear to find low carbohydrate beer quite to their liking. In the Chicagoland area where I reside, Miller Lite is the number one selling beer. Sales increases at Anheuser-Busch have been bolstered by the popularity of Bud Light, making this beer not only the number one selling low carbohydrate beer, but also the best selling beer, period, in the United States. Even Coors is in on the act, recently pushing Miller Lite out of the position as the second-best selling light beer nationally, with its Coors Light.

In Germany, where beer is virtually the national drink, brewers have even formulated great tasting *Diät Biere*, literally, diet beers, that are low in carbohydrates and brewed specifically for diabetics, in other words, a German-styled, low carbohydrate light beer. It is brewed according to the strict regulations for brewing a superior beer, known as the *Reinheitsgebot*, the beer "purity law", an ancient German brewing law that still imposes penalties for those who dare brew an insipid and adulterated beer that doesn't follow the highest standards of German beer brewing.

In the United States, where any mention of beer as a food substance is discouraged by the Bureau of Alcohol Tobacco and Firearms, the idea of marketing a low carbohydrate beer that would fit into a low carbohydrate diet, let alone be profiled as a beer for diabetics, is unthinkable.

Seems to me that the BATF might want to reevaluate their position on this. A smart beer importer ought to look at the current market of over 17 million diabetics in the U.S.A today. In addition, 1 million people, aged twenty or older, are being diagnosed with diabetes each year.

Before we get into a discussion as to the merits of low carbohydrate beer and its role in the diet, I think an explanation of its history is warranted.

Birth of Light Beer

Popular beer folklore states that the first low carbohydrate beer was formulated and marketed by New York's Rheingold Brewing Company during the mid-1960s. However, a look through the brewing trade journals of the 1930s and '40s suggest evidence that American brewers were working with the low calorie/low carbohydrate concept at least twenty-five years earlier. After the end of National Prohibition in 1933, brewers began actively courting women as potential beer drinkers. In order to sway women away from the sweet cocktails of the Prohibition-era, many American breweries reformulated their beers from the stronger and richer brews of the pre-Prohibition era and settled for lighter beers with a sweeter taste profile. Others, like the Pilsen Brewing Company in Chicago, actually advertised some of their products as *"non-fattening."* Pilsen's Yusay brand was actually promoted during the late 1930s and early '40s with the advertising tag line, *"It's The Right Weigh!"* with an ad of a smiling woman on a scale.

Articles in newspapers during this period often quoted *Braumeisters* who pointed out the low caloric features of their products. Most men probably ignored this information but they weren't the real targeted audience anyway. With the hoopla that surrounded the return of legal beer, men were rightfully accepted as the core of beer drinkers. Women, a demographic group ignored by brewers before National Prohibition, were the new targets, now to be courted by American breweries.

Rheingold's Gablinger brand tried to achieve a broader market share with more than just cute advertising, however. They actually reformulated their flagship brand (if you can call it "reformulated") in 1967 by adding water to their full-strength beer. No one was fooled by this bit of brewing chicanery, neither women nor an emerging new segment of beer drinkers, health and sport enthusiasts.

In short time, the age of sugar free, low calorie and low carbohydrate food items was upon us, not only in the beer industry but also in the food and soda pop trades.

About the same time that Gablinger was tanking in the retail market, beer scientists discovered an enzyme that could convert all the seemingly non-fermentable sugars in beer to alcohol. By converting these residual sugars to additional alcohol, the caloric and carbohydrate contents of the beer were lowered. In a final step, the additional alcohol was drawn off, leaving a product that had a fuller taste profile than a beer and water blend.

Meister Brau Lite

Meister Brau, Incorporated, once a Chicago-based regional brewery with national aspirations, quietly picked up the formula in 1966 for a low calorie/low carbohydrate beer using this new enzyme technology, with its purchase of Buckeye Brewing in Toledo, Ohio. M-B's business plan was to move beyond beer and into the world of low calorie/low carbohydrate products including candies, cookies and even a soap company called the Lite Soap Company of Aurora, Illinois. Soon after the purchase of the Buckeye Brewery and the subsequent reformulation of its light beer by M-B, Meister Brau Lite was born. A positive attribute of the beer, pushed by M-B, was the claim that Meister Brau Lite was "non-filling." The word "Lite," a cute little play on the word "light," was born into the world of American beer, lifted from a bar of soap. The beer and the word "Lite" would become Meister Brau's two most valuable assets.

Unfortunately, Meister Brau's attempt to bring M-B Lite beyond its regional constrictions plus its financially-draining involvement with non-brewing enterprises, proved to be too much for this innovative Chicago brewery.

Lite Beer from Miller

In 1972, the beleaguered Meister Brau, Incorporated sold-off most of its beer formulas, trademarks, brands and labels to Miller Brewing Company of Milwaukee. Backed by the deep pockets of parent company Phillip Morris, Incorporated and the formula for Meister Brau Lite, now known as Lite Beer from Miller, Miller began to exploit the same markets that Meister Brau had initially courted. As in the hands of M-B, Lite Beer from Miller was primarily geared towards female beer drinkers. In addition to women, the low calorie/low carbohydrate product was also targeted towards the larger market of men and the increasingly important sub-category of beer drinkers, sports and health enthusiasts.

For a while, it appeared to be a hard battle. Lite beer, and the few other low calorie/low carbohydrate beers in the retail beer market, had image problems. Not only was taste an issue, this new beer style was viewed by hardcore male beer drinkers as wimpy, a woman's drink. One industry insider took the argument a step further, actually labeling it as a *"fag"* beer. But in the emerging era of Jim Fixx and the success of his running philosophy, the increasing consumption of health foods, diet sodas and candies, Lite beer started to find an audience.

After a test marketing of Lite Beer from Miller in the blue-collar town of Anderson, Indiana, the beer tested positively. Moved to the national market, the beer continued to test well. There was, however, the lingering perception that it was a woman's drink or worse.

Enter the now familiar string of television endorsements by ex-jocks. With the amusing commercials (*"Less Filling! Taste Great!"*) as the first line of assault, Miller began relentlessly pushing Lite beer, buying unprecedented amounts of TV air time during sporting events to further the market. It was only a matter of time before Lite Beer from Miller was perceived by American male beer drinkers as a beer with balls. It became a man's drink. Health enthusiasts looked at its low calorie/low carbohydrate attributes and started to buy. Women liked it because it was promoted as *"Less Filling!"*

It would take a number of years before other breweries would jump on the low calorie/low carbohydrate beer bandwagon, including Anheuser-Busch. A-B's first entry into this new beer category was Natural Light, a beer that was soon put out to pasture as a low-cost "popular-priced" beer but still sells well today. Finally realizing the growing popularity of low calorie/low carbohydrate beers, A-B introduced Bud Light and followed Miller's approach of buying commercial TV time during major sports events and sponsoring local, regional and national sporting games. With the relentless advertising of Miller and A-B, light beer became a legitimate category of beer style. Bud Light is now the number one selling beer in the U.S.

What Beer's Right For You?

A look at the sales figures of just the leading light beers for 2002, easily confirms that low calorie/low carbohydrate beers have become an accepted beer style, controlling more than 35% of the retail beer market. I have to admit, however, that I was a bit apprehensive of adding light beers to my diet. My beer tastes tended towards the fuller taste of microbrews and imports, but the choice between two light beers at the end of a long day versus one regular beer initially made the choice an easy one. I like beer. Two beers are better than one.

This soon became a simplistic argument. Experimenting with different food and beer combinations, I concluded that beer should be enjoyed with food in a matter similar to that of wine. When I enjoy a light snack or meal, I now tend towards light bodied, low carbohydrate beers to match the food I'm eating. If the meal is a spicy dish, perhaps a bit heavy, I might reach for a regular beer, always making sure that I'm keeping within the limitations of no more than 30% of my daily carbohydrate intake as beer.

Do I have favorite brews? Sure. We all do.

Are there beers I don't like? Of course. There are some low calorie/low carbohydrate beers that I swear are based on the original Gablinger formula, but in the same sense, there are also some regular beers that I won't drink.

Will I recommend beers for your enjoyment? I have to hedge a bit here. Like any beer drinker, I have my likes and dislikes. I also realize that taste is subjective and won't foist my beer likes and dislikes upon you.

One problem as I see it, that has developed out of the beer revolution of the last twenty years or so, is beer snobbery. There's a holier-than-thou attitude that permeates some beer magazines, clubs, web sites and chat rooms, carried on the philosophies of too many beer writers and enthusiasts who look down their collective noses at all beers except all-malt, "handcrafted" beers or pricey imports. As I mentioned earlier, these were actually my favorite types of beer, but as I moved through various brands and styles of beer to accommodate my food choices and carbohydrate restrictions while developing **The Drink Beer, Get Thin Diet**, I had to question my own beer chauvinism. Beer doesn't always have to be imported or handcrafted to be good. Good beer is the beer that pleases you the most. To paraphrase an old Crosby, Stills and Nash song, *"Love the beer you're with."*

Because of my beer epiphany, I now believe that there is a beer for almost anyfood, event or occasion. At that point in **The Drink Beer, Get Thin Diet** where my choices of beer became wide open, I often found myself switching between various styles, types and brands of beer, including the higher carbohydrate craft beers, imports and standard American brews but reverting back to a light bodied, low carbohydrate beer when it seemed most appropriate for whatever dish I was enjoying.

During the Initial Phase of the diet, I originally tried to limit my beer intake to low carb beers, beers that I probably wouldn't have tasted otherwise. I enjoyed some great beers. I also found some beers I'll never try again. I soon realized, however, that limiting myself to a single style of low carb beer could be boring and would seek out regular-brewed beers that fell into the 30% carbohydrate limitation. I eventually pushed aside my first thoughts that two beers were always better than one. It was this movement between different beer types and styles, between low carbohydrate and regular beers, popular, premium and super premium priced, that I believe assured my success with the diet. Open up your beer horizons and the diet, with its huge variety of beer choices, will work for you too.

The beauty of **The Drink Beer, Get Thin Diet** is the increasing range of choices you can enjoy in food and beer as the weight melts away. If you have read any of the popular low carbohydrate diet books on the market today, they all follow a similar approach—start with a restricted intake of carbohydrates and the occasional low carb beer (if one feels the need). Eventually, as the pounds come off, the dieter is allowed to increase his or her daily carbohydrate intake, but the issue of moving on to the enjoyment of regular brewed beers as the diet progresses is never discussed. With the carbohydrate information of over 350 worldwide beers included in the listing in Chapter 6, you can open up your choices of both beer and food.

Take advantage of these choices, but don't abuse them, and one day when you're looking in the mirror, you'll discover a new you!

Chapter 4

The Diet

The Initial Phase-In order to get your metabolism switched over to an effective fat-burning machine, it is necessary to stringently quantify the amount of carbohydrates that you initially take in. This temporary restriction means **no beer**, but is necessary for the first five days of the diet while your metabolism switches over from its carbohydrate dependency. During this short period, you must limit your daily carbohydrate intake to no more than 20 grams during each of the first three days. At the end of this 72-hour period of metabolic transition, you may now move up to an intake of 25 grams of carbohydrates beginning with day four, 30 grams on day five and finally settle in with 35 grams a day during day six. Happily, at the carbohydrate intake level of 35 grams, you can now include some beer. You must remain at this 35 grams of daily carbohydrate level for a period of twenty-four days. Combined with the initial buildup from 20 to 35 grams of carbohydrates during the first six days of the diet, plus the twenty-four days at 35 grams of carbohydrates, the initial weight loss phase will last 30 days.

Days 1-3	**Day 4**	**Day 5**	**Days 6-30**
20 grams of carbs daily	25 grams of carbs daily	30 grams of carbs daily	35 grams of carbs daily with beer equaling no more than 30% of your carb intake

The Transitional Phase-Beginning with day thirty-one, you can begin the less restrictive Transitional Phase, adding an additional 5 grams of carbohydrates per week to your diet until you reach a generous daily level of 55 grams of carbohydrates a day. During the Initial Phase of the diet, you will have experienced a rapid loss in weight and inches during the first thirty days of the diet. These quick results will slow down as you begin the second part of the diet. This Transitional Phase is necessary, however. What this phase of the diet does is ready you for the final Maintenance Phase of **The Drink Beer, Get Thin Diet**. This Transitional Phase will establish the patterns for a lifetime of healthy eating, accompanied with moderate amounts of low carbohydrate and regular beer. A typical example of the weight loss to expect during the Initial and Transitional Phases follows.

Target Weight Loss—40 pounds
**Average weight loss in the Initial Phase
(first thirty days)**—20 pounds

Average weight loss during the Transitional Phase
  —2-3 pounds per week
Length of Transitional Phase—6-10 weeks

On day thirty-one, increase your carbohydrate level to 40 grams per day. Seven days later, move your carbohydrate level to 45 grams per day. The next week, move up to 50 grams of carbohydrates per day. Once you reach the 55-gram level, maintain that level of daily carbohydrates until you reach your targeted weight. Also note that your carbohydrate intake from beer also increases during the Transitional Phase from 12 grams to 16.5 grams of carbohydrates.

Remember, the time frame example above is an approximation for a typical 40-pound weight loss. If your target is less or more than my 40-pound weight loss example, the time frame will be shorter or longer.

Week 5	Week 6	Week 7	Week 8
40 grams of carbs daily with beer consisting of no more than 30% of your daily carb intake	45 grams of carbs daily with beer consisting of no more than 30% of your daily carb intake	50 grams of carbs daily with beer consisting of no more than 30% of your carb intake	55 grams of carbs daily with beer consisitng of no more than 30% of your carb intake

Once you reach Week 8, maintain this level of carbohydrate consumption daily until you reach your targeted weight.

The Maintenance Phase-Congratulations! You've reached your targeted weight. You now enter the most important phase of this diet. I'm sure, though, that most of you will consider the Initial and Transitional Phases as being the most important parts of this diet. You've lost weight and inches, hopefully have started a moderate exercise program and are really feeling good about the new you. But if you fall back to the old eating and drinking habits that made you begin this diet in the first place, your commendable efforts will be for naught. Maintenance is the key to a healthy and happy you. *It is the most important phase of* **The Drink Beer, Get Thin Diet**. Your goal during the Maintenance Phase is to finally reach a balance of your daily carbohydrate intake level equal to or greater than your daily protein level.

Protein Intake

I've been concentrating the discussion on daily carbohydrate intake, but your intake of protein is equally important. How much protein should you eat each day? My personal experience has shown that a daily protein intake of 80 to 120 grams of protein is sufficient and seems to satisfy my daily nutritional requirements. Enough evidence now indicates that a typical low fat, low protein, high carbohydrate diet can indeed lead to some weight loss. Unfortunately, much of this loss is from muscle, a dangerous situation. With adequate amounts of body building protein, you will avoid this loss in muscle mass.

During the beginning of the Maintenance Phase, increase you daily intake of carbohydrates by 5-gram increments weekly, until your daily carbohydrate level nears or equals your daily protein level. For instance, I have found that a daily intake of 100 grams of protein is enough to keep my hunger pangs at bay and feeling strong and healthy. For you, 110 or maybe 120 grams of protein might be needed to ward off hunger and feel strong and healthy. You would therefore target your daily intake of carbohydrate grams to at least match your daily protein intake. With a range of 80 to 120 grams of protein daily, you have a 40-gram range to work within.

Your protein intake depends as much on your daily level of activity and your feelings of hunger. If you lead a less physical way of life, tend towards the lower range of protein intake. If you are physically active, for instance run, bike or lift weights a few times weekly, consider your daily protein intake towards the higher level. After trial and error, I have not only increased my daily carbohydrate level to equal my daily protein level, but I have surpassed my daily protein level of 100 grams and added an additional 20 grams of carbohydrates to my diet. This gives me a balance of 100 grams protein to 120 grams of carbohydrates eaten daily. Your results might vary, but by experimentation, you will find your personal balance of protein and carbohydrates.

Although the real success of this diet can be measured by the realignment of your fat to muscle ratio, indicated by the ever loosening fit of your clothes, I also continue to monitor my weight weekly. If I see that I've gained a pound or two during the Maintenance Phase (I've been known to cheat on the diet), I immediately cut back 10 grams of carbohydrates and speed up the pace of my three-times-a-week biking routine until I return to my target weight. I then add back 5 grams and maintain this carbohydrate level for a week. At this point, I add back my final allotment of 5 grams of carbohydrates, returning to my normal daily carbohydrate level.

This weekly monitoring of weight and the balancing of protein and carbohydrates can be analogous to the fine-tuning of a carburetor. In order for the engine (your body) to run in its most efficient manner, a tiny computer chip (you) monitors the correct ratio of gasoline (protein) and air (carbohydrates) that provide the most efficient combustion (energy).

Chapter 5

A Six-Pack of Diet Strategies

Diet Tips

Tip 1. In order to keep your metabolism burning fat and to suppress any tempting hunger pangs, you must eat breakfast, lunch and dinner, supplemented with at least three snacks. If hunger continues to plague you, eat, but eat wisely. Grab a slice or two of lean meat or a couple of hard-boiled eggs and a small green salad, great standbys for stopping you from slipping off the diet. Examples of daily menus for all phases of the diet can be found in the recipe section of the book.

I've also had good success with the low carbohydrate milkshake products now on the market. Two scoops of protein powder, mixed with a cup of water, two ice cubes and a small handful of strawberries are a satisfying snack. Be careful, however, with this quick snack; some protein mixes can contain up to 24 grams of carbohydrates per serving. There are other protein powder mixes out there with much less carbohydrates so shop around. Check the Appendix for some suggestions. Remember; the diet is qualitative, not necessarily quantitative. If you find you need to increase your protein intake in order to ward off hunger, do so—just don't add unnecessary carbohydrates.

Tip 2. Your intake of fats will consist of pure fats such as butter and animal fats (remember the "French Paradox?"), olive oil, non-toasted sesame oil, peanut oil, safflower oil, hazelnut oil, sunflower oil, canola oil and almond oil. You don't have to limit your intake of these fats, but I don't suggest you try to drink a bottle of olive oil with your dinner, either. These oils will not make you fat (as long as you keep the carbohydrates under control), but will be used by your body as an energy source. Do not use margarine or diet spreads that are partially-hydrogenated (read the label). Mayonnaise is permitted.

Tip 3. Drink a minimum of 64 ounces of water a day. Water helps to pass waste from your body, a good thing. Don't think that limiting your water intake will somehow increase your weight loss. On the contrary, the more water you drink, the quicker you will lose weight. The first week you'll find yourself heading to the bathroom more often than usual. This condition will disappear as your body adjusts to the diet. I also drink a large glass of seltzer or sparking water before every 12-ounce serving of beer I consume. Not only is it good for you, it also fills you up and blunts the craving for more beer. If you don't like carbonated water, plain tap water will do just fine.

Tip 4. Alcohol interferes with the absorption of vitamins A, D and K. Although I'm not suggesting that your alcohol intake will be so extreme as to cause a vitamin problem, a daily multivitamin is still advisable. If you experience leg cramps, lightheadedness or fatigue, especially during the first week or so, take a daily potassium supplement or use any of the over-the-counter salt substitutes such as Morton's Lite Salt which has potassium chloride as an ingredient. This condition is normally a result of frequent urination during the first week of metabolic change. I experienced a general tiredness in my legs during the first week of the diet. Potassium supplements took care of this in less than a day. Also make sure you are consuming your targeted protein *and* carbohydrate levels. Cutting back on either one to increase your weight loss is not worth blowing the diet because of hunger pangs or feeling woozy.

Tip 5. Don't eat carbohydrates or drink beer unless you're taking in some protein at the same time. The combining of protein with carbohydrates helps to keep the rise in glucose levels caused by the consumption of carbohydrates and the subsequent release of insulin at a stable level. Maintain a balance. A handful or two of peanuts or a slice of salami with your beer is better than drinking a beer alone and more satisfying.

Tip 6. Restrict your beer intake to no more than 30 percent of your daily carbohydrate intake. At the 35-grams-of-carbohydrates level that is allowed daily during the Initial Phase of the diet, with a little rounding off, that means no more than 11 grams of carbohydrates in the form of beer. This initially limits you to virtually all the typical low carbohydrate beers e.g., two 12-ounce servings of Amstel Light, total of a little over 10 grams, or smaller portions of regular beer e.g., one 12-ounce serving of Budweiser, 10.6 grams, one 12-ounce serving of Redhook Hefeweissen, 10.58 grams of carbohydrates. I have to admit that my choice of low carbohydrate beer during the first weeks of the diet was based on the simple fact that I could have two of these type beers daily if I wished. This was a personal choice. If you want two low carbohydrate beers (or one 12-ounce serving of allowable regular beers) with your weekday evening meal, go right ahead.

Don't Push It!

After the Initial Phase is over and you begin the more generous Transitional Phase, your beer choices open up considerably. As you move up in 5-gram increments of carbohydrates weekly, the carbohydrates allocated for beer enjoyment also move up. At 40 grams of carbohydrates, a 30 percent allocation gives you 12 grams of carbohydrates available for beer. 45 grams gives you 13.50 grams for beer. 50 grams of carbohydrates gives you a new number of 15 grams of disposable carbohydrates for beer. At the 55-grams-of-carbohydrates level that is allowed daily during the last level of the Transitional Phase, and with 30 percent of this number rounded off to 17 grams of allowable carbohydrates in the form of beer, you can continue to enjoy a maximum of two 12-ounce servings of any low carbohydrate beer. You can also move on to one 12-ounce serving of virtually any of the regular beers or a combination of perhaps one 12-ounce serving of a low carbohydrate beer and a regular beer.

"Wait a minute," you might ask. *"A tasty Miller Lite is only 3.2 grams of carbohydrates per 12-ounce can. At 12, 13.50, 15 and finally 17 grams of allowable*

carbohydrates in the form of beer during the transitional phase of the diet, I could eventually drink up to five cans of Miller Lite and still stay under the daily carbohydrate allowance for beer."

This is an argument that comes up on a regular basis when I explain how beer fits into **The Drink Beer, Get Thin Diet**. Ah, the beer drinker's mentality! It's not enough to enjoy a beer or two with a meal and still lose weight. They always want more. I feel your pain, but it's this kind of thinking that will get you into trouble. In theory, the consumption of three, four or five cans of beer daily would be a perfectly logical assumption. There is, however, a level of moderation that must be adhered to, especially when you're trying to reach your targeted weight level. Putting aside any discussion of over consumption, binge drinking or alcohol abuse, personal experiences have shown me that any more than two beers in a day can bring down your mental diet defenses during the Transitional Phase. By the time you finish your third beer, dietary limitations and restrictions tend to melt away. Your strength to avoid temptation might be greater than those who have successfully followed this two, 12-ounce servings restriction during the Transitional Phase, but I doubt it. If you're reading this book to lose weight, I might venture to say that moderation and restraint are not your strong suits.

These little virtues have always been a struggle for me too. To be honest, there was a time or two (or three?) when I succumbed to the temptations of more than my daily allotted amount of beer while developing **The Drink Beer, Get Thin Diet**. I'd like to tell you it was because I was testing the parameters of the diet, but I'd be lying. What I did learn, however, was that you take a chance of slowing the momentum of your weight loss by pushing the limits of your daily beer consumption, especially if you also start eating high carbohydrate foods with the beer, a real no-no. So if you do sneak an extra beer in, here and there, stay with protein choices only to snack on.

However, don't lose hope with this little caveat. During the Maintenance Phase, you can, on occasion, reward yourself and increase you beer consumption to three, 12-ounce servings of low carbohydrate or even regular brewed beer.

Good things come to those who wait! The choice is yours. If you falter, get right back on track. Don't wait until tomorrow to restart the diet or Monday if you falter on the weekend.

Three Beers A Day?

During the final Maintenance Phase, with your targeted weight level now reached, you can begin to enjoy the occasional three beers a day. Many followers of **The Drink Beer Get Thin Diet** nonetheless keep their daily beer consumption down to two 12-ounce servings or less, but reward themselves on Friday nights or Saturdays with three beers. This is the loose rule of thumb that I have followed with success. After all, your weight is down to your targeted weight by now and you can begin to enjoy more flexibility in your food and drink choices.

There might be some days you just don't feel like drinking a beer or two. After a while, the novelty of actually drinking a beer on a weight reduction program usually *diminishes* the taste for a malted beverage. On the Maintenance Phase, you can even get a little crazy if you desire, perhaps substituting the carbohydrate difference of not having your daily beer allowance with a Whopper Jr.® (28 grams of carbohydrates) for lunch, or some other "forbidden" food if you like. Just remember, the consumption of beer is not necessary for success in this diet; it's just a pleasant diversion and reward to teach you moderation in both your eating and drinking habits and yet still lose weight. One of the great things about this diet is you knowing that you can have a beer or two, or three in the Maintenance Phase, and still lose weight!

Just remember to keep the total carbohydrate level of all beer consumed limited to 30 percent of all your carbohydrate consumption for the day. My personal level of carbohydrate consumption is now 120 grams per day, leaving me an allowance of 36 grams of carbohydrates in the form of beer, well within the range of many of the regular-brewed beers on the market today. This level of daily carbohydrate intake was established with a bit of trial and error. As soon as I noted a weight increase at 130 grams of daily carbohydrate intake, I pulled back to 120 grams. When I experienced no weight loss, I went back another 10 grams of carbohydrates to 110 grams. When the slight weight gain was gone, I moved up to 115 carbohydrate grams for a week and then up again to my current level of 120 grams of carbohydrates a day. At this level I have built up enough of a carbohydrate buffer to seldom go over my total carbohydrate level for the day, even if I do reach for that third beer and second piece of pizza.

By now, you should realize that you have to remain vigilant in what you eat and drink and how much, even after you've reached your targeted weight level. After a while, however, the constant reinforcement of checking the carbohydrate level of the food and beer you consume becomes almost intuitive. However, don't take anything for granted. If you're unsure of the carbohydrate content of any food item or beer, check a carbohydrate listing. When in doubt, leave it out.

A Final Thought

If you look hard enough for faults in **The Drink Beer, Get Thin Diet**, you'll probably find one. As I mentioned earlier, a close friend who tried the diet moaned for weeks about drinking low carbohydrate beer during the Initial Phase of the diet. When I pointed out that there were a number of regular beers that fell within the carbohydrate limitations of the Initial and Transitional Phases, he admitted I was right. Now 30 pounds lighter, he nonetheless swears that Amstel Light is as good as its big brother, the higher-carbohydrate Heineken.

Even my wife gave me hell during the first month of the diet. *"You're crazy!"* she said. *"It was steak last night, bacon and eggs this morning and now beer boiled shrimp dipped in butter? And how many beers did you have tonight?"*

In one month I went from a size 48 pants to a 44. I dropped 25 pounds. Now I have to buy twice as much beer because my wife is also on the diet. I joke about this wifely episode when I tell friends about the diet, but I'm glad she joined me. Embark on the diet with a friend or loved one for support and encouragement, someone you can call, talk to or share a beer with if you ever start to waiver. Everybody needs a drinking buddy!

I guarantee you'll meet more people while on this diet who will laugh when you tell them the basic premise of **The Drink Beer, Get Thin Diet**. With some people, you'll argue about the simple logic and enjoyable aspects of the diet until you're blue in the face but they'll always have a rebuttal. Don't waste your time arguing the merits of this diet adventure with the non-believers; let your weight loss do your talking!

Chapter 6

List of Beer Carbohydrate Levels
Serving Size = 12-ounces Unless Indicated Otherwise
Carbohydrates in Grams

The following beer carbohydrate counts have been provided by cooperating breweries throughout the United States, Canada, Australia, New Zealand and Europe. These figures should be used as flexible guidelines only. Breweries can and do reformulate their brews on occasion, but usually not in significant measures. However, there might be very old or very recent beer carbohydrate numbers that are in the public domain that are slightly different than those listed below. Some breweries only bottle their beers in 750 ml containers versus the typical American 355 ml bottles and cans. The carbohydrate listing for these larger bottles have been figured at the smaller 355 ml, or 12-ounce size unless noted otherwise. Please also note that the states of Utah, Colorado, Kansas, Oklahoma and certain counties restrict the alcoholic content of beer sold in their areas. These beers are referred to in the following list as 3.2 (%). Coors also uses the term "Repeal" to indicate a full strength beer. I will continue to update the carbohydrate listings of beer products from cooperating breweries on our web site, http://www.DrinkBeerGetThinDiet.com.

Some breweries were amazingly cooperative in providing carbohydrate information for all their products, including Anheuser-Busch, Miller, Coors and Pabst. But for every single brewery offering nutritional analysis information of their products, there were ten others that either chose to ignore my inquires or could not provide relevant information. Current Bureau of Alcohol, Tobacco and Firearms regulations do not require a nutritional analysis (calories, carbohydrates, protein and fat) of beer produced or imported into the United States on their containerized products (bottles, cans, etc.) unless they are indicated as being "light" or "lite". Their explanation is as follows;

"On August 10, 1993, the Bureau of Alcohol, Tobacco and Firearms (ATF) published an advanced notice of proposed rulemaking (ANPRM) in the Federal Register soliciting comments from the public and industry on whether the regulations should be amended to require nutritional information on labels of alcohol beverages.

The comment period for the ANPRM closed on February 7, 1994. ATF received 55 comments in response to the advance notice. Only 7 of these comments came from consumers. However, 5 of the 7 consumers who commented opposed nutrition labeling. Overall, 80 percent of the comments received in response to the ANPRM opposed nutrition labeling for alcohol beverages. Thirty-five of the comments opposing nutrition labeling were submitted on behalf of industry, both domestic and foreign.

After careful consideration of the petition and the comments received in response to the advance notice, ATF determined that an amendment of the regulations to provide nutrition information on labels of alcohol beverages is unnecessary and unwarranted."

Could a brewery voluntarily add carbohydrate or caloric information to all their containerized products if they wanted to? Probably, but the cost of redesigning labels and cans to reflect an average analysis of all their products could place an undue financial burden on marginally profitable breweries wanting to sell their products in the U.S., and since the BATF feels that "...*nutrition information on labels* [and cans] *is unnecessary and unwarranted"*, don't expect to find carbohydrate information, or any nutritional information, on regular brewed beers.

"In reviewing its position, the Bureau has found that specifying the caloric content of the product in comparison to the brewer's regular product is no longer essential to give the consumer a point of reference. Also, the Bureau has determined that carbohydrate references should be handled in the same manner as caloric references."

Of course, because light beers are lower in carbohydrates and calories than their regular products, the brewers are forced to add this information and an average nutritional analysis to their bottles, cans and advertising to confirm to BATF regulations and as a sales inducement for those trying to restrict carbohydrate or calorie intake.

"The Bureau will not sanction any caloric or carbohydrate references on labels that do not contain a statement of average analysis."

The more savvy brewers, however, have made complete nutritional analyses of all their products and offer this information to anyone who wants to know what they're drinking through handouts and product spec sheets.

I was initially disappointed, however, that many of the breweries that could not provide this information were the smaller sized microbreweries that are struggling to make an impact in the national beer market. Some of these breweries took the approach that their products were brewed for their taste, not for their nutritional aspects. But quite often, a check of their web sites would reveal the standard general argument that beer contains vitamins and minerals, implying a nutritional benefit. You can't have it both ways.

Another small brewery left me shaking my head after my inquiry for the carb content of their products. *"We don't list the IBU's, calories, carbs, etc...for any of our brews. Unless it's a special circumstance."* I was going to reply that a customer inquiry for information on the nutritional analysis of their products certainly seemed like a special circumstance but figured I'd get nowhere with that argument. The reluctance or inability by some breweries to provide information on what I'm putting into my body is somewhat unnerving. The BATF suggest that those interested in finding out what's in the beer they drink *"...should contact the company by writing to the address on the label. Most companies will assist you if you ask them for this information."*

Good luck here. My initial research had already indicated that a good number of smaller breweries wouldn't assist me with information on the nutritional analysis of their products. But in the last two years or so since I began accumulating the carbohydrate contents of as many beers as possible for this book, a remarkable trend has begun. More breweries than ever, including a number of smaller sized and regional ones, are now providing nutritional analysis specifications of their products.

I suspect a lot of this new found willingness is the growing recognition that low carbohydrate diets are more popular than ever. Beer sales in the U.S. have been flat for years so anything that can stimulate additional growth in the industry is important to brewers.

Anheuser-Busch, with the launching of its new Michelob Ultra, leaves no doubt as to whom this beer, with a carbohydrate content of only 2.6 grams, is targeted towards. *"We pride ourselves on watching consumer trends,"* says Anheuser-Busch senior brand manager Anne Suppinger. She said extensive research shows a surprising number of beer drinkers watch their carbohydrates.

Adds one retailer about Ultra fitting into a low carb diet, *"I'm selling more (Michelob Ultra) than any of the other flavors except regular. Obviously, some are regular Michelob drinkers who are carbohydrate-conscious people on high protein, low carb diets. I'm not on the floor all the time, but of the people I've seen with it in their carts, it's men and women who are a little bit older, 35-plus."*

I also wouldn't accept explanations from some breweries that gave me carbohydrate ranges of their products. If I couldn't get specifics on carbohydrate counts from these breweries, I found it hard to accept their estimates of carbohydrates in their products. A look at the wide disparity of carbohydrates in the products of the Boston Beer Company, for instance, shows exactly what I mean with their Spring Ale coming in at 16.53 grams of carbohydrates per 12-ounce serving versus their Double Bock at 32.40 grams. To try to "guesstimate" carbohydrate contents of beer styles or *"...typical microbrewed beers..."* as one brewery tried to argue, could be the difference between success or failure on **The Drink Beer, Get Thin Diet**.

I also heard from one famous Canadian and one equally famous Japanese brewery, both of which refused my request for a product analysis of their beers, both claiming proprietary information. With so many breweries freely offering carbohydrate information for publication in this book, I found their refusal for carbohydrate information of their products to be peculiar, if not somewhat paranoid.

Diabetics might also find the carbohydrate listings of beer useful. A reading of current literature and a check of numerous web sites that offer support to those with Type I and Type II diabetes are vague and often incorrect with their assumptions of the carbohydrate content of beer. Here is a small table from the web site of a nationwide diabetes center listing the average carbohydrate content of beer:

Beverage	**Amount**	**Calories**	**Carbohydrates**
Regular beer	12-ounces	150	14 grams
Light beer	12-ounces	100	6 grams
NA beer	12-ounces	50	10 grams

Compare this chart of average carbohydrate contents to the extensive listed values of carbohydrates in beer that were provided by over sixty worldwide breweries. In today's beer revolution, there is no such thing as a "typical" beer. To list all regular beers as containing 12 grams of carbohydrates per 12-ounce serving is misleading and potentially harmful to those individuals who have to control their carbohydrate intake and blood glucose levels. Even worse is the typical carbohydrate count given for non-alcoholic beers. The variance between products can be extreme, e.g. A-B's Busch NA at 12.90, O' Doul's Amber at 18.00 and Beck's Hacke NA at 20.00 grams of carbohydrates per 12-ounce serving.

I would suggest to those breweries that have not done a full nutritional analysis of their beers and those that hold their information as proprietary, are ignoring the 6% of the United States population that suffers from diabetes. Almost another 1 million people will be diagnosed with diabetes this year. A sizable portion of this group can still drink beer but drink mostly low carbohydrate beers, simply because the carbohydrate content of only these products lists a product analysis breakdown on the container.

If you are diabetic and your doctor allows the moderate consumption of beer with food, the following carbohydrate listings of beer can be an invaluable guide to enjoying moderate amounts of regular-brewed beers.

The final decision of whether to drink alcohol as a person suffering from diabetes and what to drink, lies with you. It remains essential that, if you wish to include beer in your diet, you consult your doctor. With certain diabetes medications, drinking increases the risk of hypoglycemia, so be aware.

Please note: The following information is provided as a general guide of beer and carbohydrate levels for those wishing to follow a low carbohydrate approach to dieting and sufferers of diabetes. It is not a substitute for specific advice from your General Practitioner.

If you can't find your favorite brew among those listed below and would like to include it in the diet, I would suggest you call your favorite brewery and ask if they can provide you with relevant carbohydrate information or simply switch to one of the fine brands listed here. Don't forget to check our web site at http://www.DrinkBeerGetThinDiet.com for beer carbohydrate updates.

Amstel

Amstel	10.65
Bock	17.75
Gold	14.20
Lentebock	17.74
Light	5.33

Meibock	17.75
Malt	21.30
Oud Bruin	19.52
1870	12.42

Anchor

Anchor Steam	16.00

Anheuser-Busch

Budweiser	10.60
Budweiser 3.2	8.70
Bud Light	6.60
Bud Light 3.2	5.20
Bud Ice	9.00
Bud Ice Light	5.20
Bud Ice Light 3.2	3.60
Bud Dry	7.80
Bud Dry 3.2	6.30
Michelob	13.00
Michelob 3.2	12.20
Michelob Light	11.70
Michelob Light 3.2	9.30
Michelob Ultra	2.90
Michelob Golden Draft	12.90
Michelob Golden Draft 3.2	10.50
Michelob Golden Draft Light	7.00
Michelob Golden Draft Light 3.2	5.50
Michelob Dry	7.90
Michelob Classic Dark	14.50

Michelob Amber Bock	14.50
Michelob Amber Bock 3.2	11.90
Michelob Hefeweizen	18.40
Michelob Hefeweizen 3.2	11.90
Michelob Porter	20.20
Michelob Pale Ale	16.70
Michelob Honey Lager	17.90
Michelob Honey Lager 3.2	14.90
Michelob Black & Tan	16.30
Red Wolf	11.70
Red Wolf 3.2	9.20
O'Doul's	15.00
O'Doul's Amber	18.00
Busch	10.00
Busch 3.2	8.10
Busch NA	12.90
Busch Light	6.70
Busch Light 3.2	5.20
Busch Ice	13.20
Busch Ice 3.2	10.30
Natural Light	6.60
Natural Light 3.2	5.30
Natural Ice	9.40
Natural Ice 3.2	7.60
King Cobra	15.40
Hurricane	9.40
Tequiza	9.10
Tequiza 3.2	8.10
ZeigenBock	14.40

August Schell

August Schell Light Beer	4.00

Beck's

Beck's	10.00
Beck's Dark	11.00
Beck's Light	6.10
Beck's Oktoberfest	9.00
Hacke Beck NA	20.00
St. Pauli Girl	8.70
St. Pauli Girl NA	23.00

Big Rock Brewery

All Brands	12.70

Bitburger

Pils	9.05
Light	7.10
Drive NA	20.59
Koestritzer	9.94
Kandi	35.50

Bochkarev

Export	13.49
Light	13.49

Strong	21.30
Barreled	9.94
Wheat Special	15.98
Non-Alcoholic	21.66

Boddington

Boddington	12.78

Boston Beer Company

Boston Lager	19.56
Summer Ale	15.85
Octoberfest	18.72
Winter Lager	21.25
White Ale	16.86
Boston Ale	19.90
Honey Porter	20.57
Cream Stout	23.94
Cherry Wheat	16.86
Golden Pilsner	15.68
Scotch Ale	24.96
Double Bock	32.04
Cranberry Lambic	20.91
Spring Ale (Kolsch)	16.53
Hardcore Cider	19.00

Brand

Dubbelbock	17.75
Imperator	14.20

Meibock	14.20
Oud Bruin	7.10
Pilsner	10.65
Sylvester	17.75
UP	12.43
Vos	14.20
Wieckse Witte	12.42

Budweiser Budwar (aka Checkvar)

Budwar Free (NA)	9.23
Budejovicky Budwar (10%)	13.49
Budejovicky Budwar (12%)	14.42
Bud Super Strong (16%)	16.45

Caledonian Brewery

125	12.60
Burke & Hare	13.49
Burns Ale	14.35
Calders 70/-	9.45
Calders 80/-	10.50
Calders Cream	12.07
Calders Light	11.72
Caley 80/-	13.16
Golden Promise	13.85
Burns Ale	14.56
Grand Slam	12.78
IPA	12.43
Summer Ale	9.59
Festival	12.07

Mellow Yellow	12.43
Space Odessy	10.30

Carlsberg

Light	7.81
Lager	9.94
Red	10.30
Red Elephant	11.72
Elephant Malt Liquor	14.20

Carolina Beer & Beverage, LLC

Carolina Light	2.00
Charleston Wheat	5.00

Corona

Light	5.00

Clausthaler

Premium Non-Alcohol	20.60

Cooper's

Genuine Draught	7.02
Lite	4.50
Sparkling Ale	7.56
Stout	10.80

Pale Ale	5.94
Premium	11.52
Export	11.16
Dry	6.84

Coors

Artic Ice Repeal	8.98
Artic Ice 3.2	6.66
Artic Ice Export	5.82
Blue Moon Belgian White	12.87
Blue Moon Honey Blond Repeal	19.72
Blue Moon Nut Brown Repeal	16.78
Blue Moon Raspberry Repeal	20.92
Castlemaine XXXX Repeal	9.41
Coors Repeal	11.79
Coors 3.2	9.54
Coors Export	10.68
Coors Light Repeal	4.32
Coors Light 3.2	4.12
Coors Light Export	3.98
Coors Dry Repeal	5.92
Coors Dry	4.84
Cutter	15.65
Cutter Export	15.28
Extra Gold Repeal	11.65
Extra Gold 3.2	9.35
Extra Gold Export	10.58
Herman Joseph Repeal	12.21

Crooked River Brewing Company

Crooked River Expansion Draft	13.00
Crooked River Select Lager	15.70

Foster's

Abbotsford Invalid Stout	11.76
Cairns Draught	9.94
Carlton Black Ale	10.65
Carlton Cold Filtered Bitter	9.94
Carlton Draught	9.59
Carlton G	9.59
Carlton Light	10.65
Carlton Light NT	9.59
Carlton LJ	3.20
Carlton Mid Strength Bitter	14.20
Carlton Mid Strength Bitter QLD	14.56
Carlton Premium Dry	9.94
Cascade Bitter	9.59
Cascade Draught	9.23
Cascade Lager	9.59
Cascade Pale Ale	9.94
Cascade Premium	11.00
Cascade Premium Light	11.36
Cascade Stout	15.98
Crown Lager	11.00
Dogbolter	14.20
Fiji Bitter	9.94
Fiji Gold	5.68

Foster's Ice	11.36
Foster's Lager	11.00
Foster's Light-NZ	10.30
Foster's Light Ice	11.00
Foster's Special Bitter	12.78
Guinness Draught	12.78
Guinness	17.40
303 Ice Gold	11.76
KB Lager	11.00
Kent Old Brown	11.36
Matilda Bay Bitter	15.27
Matilda Bay Premium	12.78
Melbourne Bitter	11.00
NT Draught	9.94
Power's Bitter	9.94
Power's Gold	9.23
Power's Ice	8.88
Redback Light	9.59
Redback Original	12.78
Resch's DA	11.76
Resch's Draught	9.94
Resch's Pilsener	10.30
Resch's Pilsener (New Zealand)	8.88
Resch's Real Bitter	10.65
Resch's Real Bitter (New Zealand)	10.65
Richmond Lager	9.94
Sheaf Stout	18.82
Stella Artois	12.78
Victoria Bitter	11.00
Yatala Stripe	12.78

Bob Skilnik

Frederick Brewing Company

Crooked River Light   6.40

Grants

Scottish Ale   12.70

Grolsch

Amber   11.36
Herfstbok   15.62
Lentebok   12.07
Oud Bruin   12.78
Premium Pilsner   11.00
Special Malt   18.46
Wintarvorst   17.04
Zomergoud   11.36

Harpoon

Ale   17.00
IPA   12.00

Heineken

Eindejaars Bier   19.53
Heineken   10.65
Heineken Oud Bruin   19.70

Heineken Tarwebok	23.08
Kylian	23.08
Lingen's Blond	17.75
Vollenhoven's Stout	19.53

Highfalls Brewing Inc.

Dundee's Classic Lager	13.00
Geesse Beer	13.50
Genesse Cream Ale	15.00
Genesse Ice	12.00
Genny Light	5.50
Genesse NA	15.00
Genesse Red	14.00
12 Horse	14.00
Honey Brown Lager	13.50
Honey Brown Light	7.70
Honey Brown Light >3.2	9.30
Michael Shea's Irish Amber	13.00
Michael Shea's Black & Tan	13.00

Hudepohl-Schoenling Brewing Company

Burger Classic Beer	12.40
Burger Light	9.60
Christian Moerlein Select Lager	15.70
Christian Moerlein Bock	15.70
Hudy Delight Premium Light Beer	3.70
Little Kings Cream Ale	15.80
Hudepohl 14-K	12.40
Schoenling Lager	12.40

Labatt

Light	7.90
Regular	9.90

Leinenkugel

Honey Weiss	12.00
Northwoods Lager	15.30
Original	13.90
Red Lager	16.20
Amber Light	7.00

Lion-Nathan

1857 Bitter	10.85
Canterbury Draught	8.05
Carbine Stout	14.35
Eagle Blue	9.80
Eagle Blue Ice	9.45
Eagle Super	9.45
Emu Bitter	12.78
Emu Draft	10.85
Emu Export	10.30
Emundi	11.00
Gulf Lager	10.85
Hahn Ice	8.75
Hahn Longbrew	4.55
Hahn Premium	11.20
Hahn Premium Light	10.85

Hahn Witbier	9.94
Ice Beer	8.05
James Squire Amber Ale	14.91
James Squire Pilsener	15.98
James Squire Porter	14.91
Light Ice	6.75
Lion Brown	8.05
Lion Light Ice	6.65
Lion Red	7.70
Old Black Ale	16.10
Southwark Bitter	9.94
Southwark Black Ale	16.10
Southwark Pale Ale	9.80
Southwark Premium	10.15
Southwark Old Stout	12.60
Southwark White	10.30
Sovereign	12.07
Speight's	7.35
Speight's Old Ale	10.15
Speights Old Dark	10.30
Steinlager	8.40
Steinlager (China)	11.72
Swan Draught	10.15
Swan Gold	9.10
Swan Mid	13.65
Swan Stout	12.60
Tooheys Amber Bitter	10.85
Tooheys Blue	15.75
Tooheys Blue Ice	12.25
Tooheys Extra Dry	8.75
Tooheys Gold	10.85
Tooheys Maxim	5.68

Tooheys New	10.85
Tooheys Old	11.20
Tooheys Pils	8.91
Tooheys Red	11.72
Waikato Draught	7.10
West End 107 Pilsener	9.94
West End Draught	8.52
West End Export	9.05
West End Gold	8.17
West End Light	7.46
XXXX Bitter	8.17
XXXX DL Lager	3.55
XXXX Draught	8.17

Miller Brewing Company

Miller Genuine Draft	13.10
Genuine Draft Light	7.00
Hamm's	12.10
Hamm's Golden Draft	12.10
Hamm's Special Light	7.30
Henry Weinhard's Amber Ale	14.00
Henry Weinhard's Dark	13.10
Henry Weinhard's Hefeweizen	12.10
Henry Weinhard's Ice Ale	13.20
Henry Weinhard's Pale Ale	13.00
Henry Weinhard's Private Reserve	9.20
High Life	13.10
High Life Ice	11.00
High Life Light	7.00
Icehouse 5.5	9.80
Icehouse 5.0	8.70

Lite Ice 5.5	4.20
Magnum Malt Liquor	9.90
Meister Brau	11.40
Meister Brau Light	4.80
Mickey's	11.20
Mickey's Ice	11.80
Miller Lite	3.20
Milwaukee's Best	11.40
Milwaukee's Best Ice	7.00
Olde English 800	10.50
Old English 800 3.2	6.90
Old English 800 7.5	13.10
Olde English 800 Ice	14.30
Red Dog	14.10
Sharp's	12.10
Southpaw Light	7.10

Millstream Brewing Company

German Pilsner	14.90
Schild Brau Amber	16.80
Millstream Wheat	11.00

Murphy Brewery

Murphy's Irish Red Beer	8.82

New Belgium

1554	22.48
Abbey, per 650 ml.	15.99

Abbey Grand Cru, per 650 ml.	16.87
Blue Paddle	11.99
Fat Tire	13.66
La Folie, per 750 ml.	18.10
Porch Swing	12.49
Sunshine Wheat	11.55

New Century

Edison Light	6.6

Pabst

Augsburger Bock	17.00
Augsburger Dark	17.00
Augsburger Golden	17.00
Augsburger Red	14.00
Blatz	12.50
Blatz Light	8.30
McSorley's Ale	15.00
McSorley's Black/Tan	14.50
Old Milwaukee	12.90
Old Milwaukee Light	8.30
Old Style	9.40
Old Style Light	12.00
Pabst	12.01
Pabst Light	8.30
Pabst NA	12.00
Schaefer	12.00
Schaefer's Light	8.30
Stroh	12.00

Stroh Light   7.00

Pete's Wicked

Honey Wheat	16.30
Oktoberfest	16.50
Pub Lager	14.00
Signature Pilsner	13.90
Strawberry Blonde	13.70
Summer Brew	14.20
Wicked Ale	15.30
Winter Brew	15.30

Pilsner Urquell

Gambrinus	9.80
Pilsner Urquell	14.70

Pittsburgh Brewing Company

Iron City Light	2.90
Iron City Light Twist	2.90

Primus

Adler	16.73
Charles Quint	25.76
Primus	13.55
Tongerlo Blonde 6	20.09
Tongerlo Brune 6	19.18

Tongerlo Triple 8	13.37

Redhook

ESB	13.90
Rye	11.95
Black Hook Porter	11.52
Ballard Bitter (IPA)	11.91
Hefeweissen	10.58
Winter Hook (Seasonal Variations)	16.00-20.00
Double Black Stout	21.13

Sarapul's

Isetskoe	20.59
Moskovskoe	19.17
Leningradskoe	27.34
Porter	29.47
Martovskoe	22.01
Rizhskoe	17.04
Zhigulevskoe	17.04
Dvoinoe Zolotoe	20.59
Sarapulskoe	20.59

Sierra Nevada

Pale Ale	16.00
Pale Bock	20.00
Porter	18.00

Spoetzl Brewery

Shiner Blond	13.00
Shiner Bock	12.90
Shiner Honey Wheat	14.50
Shiner Summer Stock	10.50
Shiner Winter Ale	17.80

Steinlager

Steinlager	8.52
Steinlager (China)	11.72

Straub

Straub	10.10
Straub Light	7.16

Warsteiner

Premium Fresh	12.78
Premium Light	8.16
Premium Verum	10.60

Widmer Brothers

Doppelbock	20.80
Hefe	13.20
HopJack	14.80

Oktoberfest	15.10
Sommerbrau	10.20
SpringFest (Alt)	13.60
Sweet Betty	10.80
Widberry	13.00
Wildwood Hard Cider	21.80

Young's

Chocolate Stout	16.80
Dirty Dicks	10.50
Export Lager	7.70
Oatmeal Stout	16.80
Old Nick	35.70
Ram Rod	12.25
Special London Ale	19.25
Winter Warmer	18.20

Yuengling Brewery

Premium	12.00
Light	6.60
Ale	10.00
Porter	14.00
Lager	12.00
Black & Tan	14.00

Chapter 7

List of Protein & Carbohydrate Levels in Food

Protein Foods

You're allowed 80 to 120 grams of protein per day, divided between three meals and three snacks. Some dieters start at the 80-gram level and play it by ear whether to raise their protein level or not. It might be a good idea to leave yourself a buffer zone in case you get hungry during the day or get a late night craving. As mentioned earlier, if you are physically active or are planning on an exercise program during the diet, you'll probably tend towards the higher end of the protein intake range.

Protein Guidelines

1 ounce of meat, fish or poultry equals 7 grams of protein

1 whole egg equals 6 grams of protein, egg white (minus yolk) equals 4 grams of protein

1 ounce of hard cheese equals 6 to 7 grams of protein (read package label for exact number)

1 ounce of soft cheese equals 3 to 4 grams of protein (read package label for exact number)

1 ounce of curd cheese equals 7 grams of protein per ¼ cup (read label for exact number)

1 ounce of tofu equals 10 grams of protein (read package label for exact number)

12-ounces of beer vary on protein content but is usually insignificant. I ignored this minor protein intake.

Poultry	Meat	Fish
Any & All	Any & All	Any & All including shellfish
Eggs	**Cheese**	**Beer**
Any & All	No more than 4 ounces daily	No more than 30% of your daily carbohydrate intake

Carbohydrate Counter for Basic Foods

As you go through the following charts, you'll begin to see how simple **The Drink Beer, Get Thin Diet** really is. Simply divide your protein allowance of 80 to 120 grams between three meals and three snacks, complimented by your daily carbohydrate allowance. The following charts only highlight a limited range of fruits, vegetables, breads, grains, cereals and more. A complete listing of carbohydrates for all foods is beyond the scope of this book but available at any bookstore or you local library. Check the Appendix for recommendations.

Fiber is an important part of carbohydrates that adds bulk to your stool and improves bowel function. It is, however, not metabolized by your body and simply passed out. Therefore, you can subtract the amount of fiber in grams from your daily carbohydrate gram intake. This is your true carbohydrate intake value. For instance, one cup of fresh strawberries has a carbohydrate content of 10 grams. It also has 4 grams of fiber. Subtracting 4 grams of fiber from 10 grams of carbohydrates leaves you with 6 grams of available carbohydrates. This is the true carbohydrate amount that you need to concern yourself with when adding up your daily carbohydrate intake. It's almost like cheating!

All carbohydrates listed here have been adjusted for fiber content. For canned or frozen goods, simply use the nutritional value information on the container for the true carbohydrate value, subtracting the fiber content in grams per serving from the carbohydrate gram content.

Vegetables

For most canned and frozen varieties, check container label.

	Size	Carbs
alfalfa seeds, sprouted, raw	1 cup.	1
artichoke, globe, fresh boiled	1 medium	13
arugula	½ cup	trace
asparagus, fresh, raw	10 spears	4

Avacado	1 medium	15
bamboo shoots, cooked	½ cup	1
beets, boiled	½ cup	6.9
beets, greens	½ cup	4
bok-choy, raw	½ cup	1
broccoli, boiled, chopped	1 cup	4
brussel sprouts, boiled	½ cup	4
butternut squash, baked	½ cup	9.5
cabbage, raw	½ cup	1.1
carrot, raw	½ cup	5
cauliflower, raw	½ cup	1.2
celery, raw	½ cup	1.2
collards, boiled	½ cup	4
cucumber, sliced	½ cup	1
eggplant, boiled	1 cup	5
fava beans	½ cup	3
fennel bulb, raw	½ cup	3.2
green beans, boiled	½ cup	3.8
lettuce, bibb, Boston	1 head, 5" diameter	2.5
iceberg	1 head, 6" diameter	4
mung beans, sprouted	1 oz.	1
mushrooms, buttons, raw	½ cup	1.1
enoki, raw	½ cup	2
oyster, raw	½ cup	1
shiitake, raw	1 oz.	3.2
mustard greens, raw	1 ½ cups	4.5
okra, raw	½ cup	3.8
olives, Calamata	1 oz	4
green, pitted	10 large	1
onion, raw	½ cup	5.6
green	½ cup	2.5

peas, edible podded, raw	½ cup	3.4
peppers, chili, raw, w/o seeds	½ cup	3.5
sweet, raw	½ cup	2.4
pimento	1 tblsp	1
potato, baked w/o skin	¼ medium	7.8
boiled w/o skin	¼ medium	6.3
radish	½ cup	1
refried beans	½ cup	10
rhubarb, boiled	½ cup	3.5
rutabaga, boiled	½ cup	6.6
sauerkraut	½ cup	5.1
spaghetti squash	½ cup	3
spinach	1 cup	1
tomatillo, raw	2 medium	4
tomato, fresh	1 medium	4.1
turnips, boiled	1 cup	4.4
water chestnuts, raw	¼ cup	7.4
wax beans	½ cup	2.3
yams, baked, boiled	¼ cup	9.4

Fruits

apple, raw	¼ apple	4.5
apricot, raw	1 medium	2.3
blackberries, raw	½ cup	5.9
blueberries, raw	½ cup	6.9
cantaloupe, raw	½ cup	5.7
cherries	5	5.1
cranberries, raw	1/3 cup	4
grapefruit	¼ whole	4.4
grapes, seedless	1/3 cup	5.3

honeydew, raw	¼ cup	3.9
kiwi	½ medium	4.4
lemon	1 medium	5.4
lime	1 medium	6.5
mango	¼ cup	8.3
orange	½ medium	5.5
peach	½ medium	4.2
pear	¼ medium	5.2
pineapple, fresh	¼ cup	4.3
raspberries	½ cup	4.2
strawberries	½ cup	3
tangerine	½ medium	4.7
watermelon	½ cup	5.5

Bread, Cereal & Grain Products

Bagel	½	15
bread, light	1 slice	8
English muffin	½	13
grain cakes (rice, popcorn, etc.)	1	7
pasta, cooked	¼ cup	10
popcorn	3 cups	8
puffed corn	1 cup	15
puffed rice	1 cup	18
puffed wheat	1 cup	18
rice, brown, cooked	¼ cup	10.4
white, cooked	¼ cup	10.2
wild, cooked	¼ cup	8.8
tortilla, corn	1	7
flour	1	11

Chapter 8

Smart Snacking

As mentioned earlier, three snacks are allowed along with three meals daily. Snacking will keep you from getting hungry between meals. It's important, however, not to let this part of the diet get away from you. Just like your daily beer allowance, careless and indiscriminate snacking can slow down your progress. In spite of the fact that **The Drink Beer, Get Thin Diet** is so liberal in what you can eat and drink, some dieters will try to push the envelope and, as a result, take in too many carbohydrates for the day.

Be sure to check the serving sizes of snacks. If a serving size, for instance, is two items or forty pieces or one cup, measure or count out the serving. Don't guess. Don't estimate. Also remember to take in protein while eating your snack. A couple of cups of popcorn without a slice or two of turkey or salami will slow your progress. Don't forget a beer with your little food respite.

As with my weakness with dessert items, uncontrolled snacking might be the ruination of many of you. Smart snacking, however, can be an important part of **The Drink Beer, Get Thin Diet** that can help you through any possible hunger pangs and cravings between meals. A snack between breakfast and lunch, lunch and dinner and even dinner and bedtime can keep you alert and feeling satisfied.

Unlike low calorie diets that give you the unexciting options of carrot sticks or celery to stave off hunger, this diet opens up an unbelievable choice of food options. The following list is from my local supermarket. Most of these brands are sold nationwide and substitutes are surely available. Check the nutritional chart on the package if you have any doubts. There is an amazing array of prepared low carbohydrate food items on the market today. It might be worth it to wander the aisles of your supermarket using the handy snack list below and see what your local food store has to offer.

Don't be put off by some of the higher-carbohydrate snack items listed here. At first glance, you might question the wisdom of eating a snack with 20 + grams of carbohydrates. Always look at the serving size. If the serving size is 50 pieces of this or 3 cups of that, for example, downsize the serving size so you can enjoy a wider variety of snacks.

Remember however, you don't have to get fancy with snacking. A slice of boiled ham with a piece of cheese and a dab of spicy mustard is just as satisfying as any of the snacks below. A small leftover portion of an entrée works just as well.

Fiber has been factored into the following carbohydrate counts.

Next Saturday, when you're sitting on the couch relaxing by the fire or enjoying the warm summer breezes on your patio, have a beer and a handful or two of some of these smart snacks listed below and think about all those poor low calorie dieters that are forcing down their "rabbit food."

Corn Chips

Brand	Serving Size	Protein	Carbs
Frito			
Original Corn Chips	32 chips	2g	14g
Scoops	11 chips	2g	11g

Crackers

Kavali			
Crispy Thin	3 pieces	1g	11g
Keebler			
Corn Bread Crackers	2 crackers	1g	11g
Toasted Buttercrisp	5 crackers	1g	10g
Toasted Onion	5 crackers	1g	10g
Toasted Sesame	5 crackers	1g	10g
Toasted Wheat	5 crackers	1g	11g
Nabisco			
Chicken in a Basket Flavor Crisp	12 crackers	2g	16g
Sociables	7 crackers	1g	9g
Original Premium Saltines	5 crackers	1g	10g
Original Thin Crisps	15 crackers	3g	20g
Premium with Multigrain	5 crackers	1g	10g

Brand	Serving Size	Protein	Carbs
Pepperidge Farm			
Ritz Crackers	5 crackers	1g	10g
Goldfish Crackers			
American Cheese	55 pieces	4g	18g
Original	55 pieces	3g	18g
Parmesan	60 pieces	4g	18g
Pizza	55 pieces	3g	18g
Pretzel	43 pieces	3g	21g
Ry Krisp			
Natural	2 crackers	2g	9g
Sesame	2 crackers	2g	8g
Stella D'Oro			
Original	1 stick	1g	6g
Sesame	1 stick	1g	6g
Wasa			
Fiber Rye	1 slice	1g	5g
Hearty Rye	1 slice	1g	7g
Light Rye	1 slice	1g	5g
Multi Grain	1 slice	2g	9g
Whole Wheat	1 slice	2g	10g

Meats, Salamis

Brand **Bridgeford**	Serving Size	Protein	Carbs
Garlic Summer Sausage	2 oz	9g	0g
Hard Salami	1 oz	6g	0g
Italian Salami	1 oz	6g	0g
Pepperoni	1 oz	6g	0g
Smoked Beef Salami	2 oz	10g	0g

Busseto

	Serving Size	Protein	Carbs
Salami Herbs de Provence	1 oz	7g	1g
Salami Picante	1 oz	7g	1g

Peanuts

Brand **Planter's**	Serving Size	Protein	Carbs
Cashew Halves	40 pieces	6g	4g
Cocktail Peanuts	5 pieces	7g	3g
Dry Roasted Peanuts	39 pieces	7g	4g
Dry Roasted Sunflower Seeds	¼ cup	7g	2g

Popcorn

Brand	Serving Size	Protein	Carbs
O-Ke-Doke			
Buttery Popcorn	3 cups	2g	12g
Cheese Flavored	2 cups	2g	11g
White Popcorn	2 1/3 cups	2g	11g
Orville Redenbacher			
Butter Popcorn	4 cups	2g	11g
Cheddar Butter	3 cups	2g	9g
Movie Theater	4 cups	2g	11g

Pretzels

Brand	Serving Size	Protein	Carbs
Manischewitz			
Bagel Pretzels	4 pretzels	3g	21g
Jays			
Fat-Free Thins	14 pretzels	3g	23g
Rold Gold			
Classic Style Fat-Free	17 pretzels	2g	22g
Tiny Twists	18 pretzels	3g	22g

Spreads

Brand	Serving Size	Protein	Carbs

Aloutte Spreadable Cheese

Brand	Serving Size	Protein	Carbs
Garlic et Herbes	2 tbsp	1g	1g
Light Garlic et Herbes	2 tbsp	2g	1g
Spinach Florentine	2 tbsp	1g	1g
Sundried Tomato et Basil	2 tbsp	1g	1g
Vegetable Jardin	2 tbsp	1g	1g

Athenos

Brand	Serving Size	Protein	Carbs
Black Olive Hummus	2 tbsp	2g	5g
Original Hummus	2 tbsp	2g	4g
Pesto Hummus	2 tbsp	2g	4g
Roasted Eggplant Hummus	2 tbsp	2g	3g
Roasted Red Pepper Hummus	2 tbsp	2g	5g
Spicy Three Pepper Hummus	2 tbsp	2g	4g

Fabrique Delices

Brand	Serving Size	Protein	Carbs
Pate De Campagne w/Black Pepper	2 oz	8g	2g

Bob Skilnik

Brand	Serving Size	Protein	Carbs
Fleur de Lait			
Mediterranean Olive	2 tbsp	2g	2g
Minced Garlic & Herbs	2 tbsp	2g	3g
Spinach Artichoke	2 tbsp	2g	2g
Kraft Cream Cheese			
Chive & Onion	2 tbsp	2g	1g
Garden Vegetable	2 tbsp	1g	1g
Pineapple	2 tbsp	1g	4g
Strawberry	2 tbsp	1g	5g
Meza			
Baked Brie in Pastry	2 tbsp	4g	4g
Baked Brie in Pastry w/Roasted Garlic	2 tbsp	4g	4g
Baked Brie w/Portabella Mushrooms & Carmelized Onions	2 tbsp	3g	4g

Nabisco

Brand	Serving Size	Protein	Carbs
Easy Cheese, Nacho (Squirt Can)	2 tbsp	5g	3g
Easy Cheese, Sharp Cheddar (Squirt Can)	2 tbsp	5g	3g

Oscar Mayer
Authentic

Braunschweiger	2 oz	8g	1g
Sandwich Spread	2 oz	4g	9g

Old Wisconsin
Original Spreadable

Pate	2 oz	8g	3g
Onion & Parsley	2 oz	8g	3g

Owl's
Cheddar Cheese

Spread	2 tbsp	3g	4g
Horseradish Cheese Spread	2 tbsp	3g	4g
Peppers Galore Cheese Spread	2 tbsp	3g	4g

Prelude
Baked Brie

en Croute	1 oz.	5g	4g

Nutritional Chart

Familiarize yourself with the chart on this page. Similar information can be found on all prepared foods. This chart was taken from a package of frozen berries. You will not find this information on fresh fruits, vegetables or meats.

Nutrition Facts

Serving Size 8 medium berries (147g)

Amount Per Serving

Calories 45	Calories from Fat 0

	% Daily Value**
Total Fat 0g*	0%
Saturated Fat 0g	0%
Cholesterol 0mg	0%
Sodium 0mg	0%
Total Carbohydrate 12g	4%
Dietary Fiber 4g	15%
Sugars 8g	
Protein 1g	

Vitamin A 0%	•	Vitamin C 160%
Calcium 2%	•	Iron 4%

*Contain less than 0.5g of fat per 140g strawberries.

**Percent Daily Values are based on a 2,000 calorie diet. Your daily values may be higher or lower depending on your calorie needs:

	Calories:	2,000	2,500
Total Fat	Less than	65g	80g
Sat Fat	Less than	20g	25g
Cholesterol	Less than	300mg	300mg
Sodium	Less than	2,400mg	2,400mg
Total Carbohydrate		300g	375g
Dietary Fiber		25g	30g

Calories per gram:
Fat 9 • Carbohydrate 4 • Protein 4

A careful look at any nutritional chart will show you the carbohydrate, fiber and protein content of the labeled product.

Chapter 9

Recipes & Menus

The focus of this recipe section is to provide you with a solid base for great tasting low carbohydrate dishes and to spark your own recipe inventiveness. As such, the recipes here are limited. Most of the recipes are based on higher carbohydrate laden recipes and adjusted to conform to the principles of a low carbohydrate diet. Refer to the Appendix for recommendations for locating low carbohydrate cookbooks.

Remember, if you're short on time, a quick hamburger patty or homemade tuna salad will do just fine. A few of the larger supermarkets in our neighborhood offer whole baked chickens to go. With the chicken, I usually heat up a can of green beans, make a simple side salad, and follow this quick and simple dinner up with some strawberries and cream for dessert. I also try to take advantage of the many frozen prepared foods on the market today such as chicken strips, fish fillets and cooked shrimp. Look in the fresh and frozen food section of your local supermarket. Food manufacturers Louis Rich and Tyson have a number of precooked time savers in the meat section of today's supermarkets including Southwestern-style chicken breast strips, beef tips with gravy and whole cooked chickens. Hormel even has a prepared meat loaf with tomato sauce that can be warmed up in minutes. Armed for the week with an arsenal of food time savers, you can try your creative hand during the weekend with some of the more sophisticated recipes in this section. During the work week, I try to keep it simple. So should you.

Don't forget the beer! I've supplied numerous recipes for dishes that just call out for a cold beer accompaniment. These dishes would be unheard of with a low calorie diet but fit quite nicely with the philosophy of **The Drink Beer, Get Thin Diet**. As an added bonus, a number of these recipes even include beer as an ingredient.

One of the criticisms of low carbohydrate diets is the redundancy of entrees or the use of recipes that are time savers but uninspiring in content. Dieting or not, it can become easy to fall into the pattern of cooking the same quick entrées because you're tired or rushed for time. The use of frozen and/or pre-cooked items can help the dieter to save time plus add needed variety to the daily menu. To help you along with your choice of a possible recipe to follow, I've included the approximate times of preparation and cooking.

You'll also notice the symbols "I," "T" and/or "M" alongside the serving portion. Some of the recipes contain enough carbohydrates to make them off limits during the Initial Phase; others, although allowable in most cases during the Transitional Phase, should be recognized as having the potential of putting you over your daily allowable carbohydrate intake through poor meal planning. The "M" symbolizes recipes for food to be enjoyed freely during the Maintenance Phase. These recipes contain the highest amounts of carbohydrates.

Like the variety you can experience with the many beers on the market today, a good mix of different foods and different methods of preparation will keep you pumped and inspired as you lose weight and inches and experience the makings of the new you.

Appetizers

This is really one of the most versatile parts of the diet. Not only can these recipes be used as appetizers, try the leftovers as one of the three designated snacks per day. For time saving dishes, use frozen, pre-cooked items when available.

Cheese Beer Ball
Serves 12   I, T, M
Prep Time: 15 minutes, Refrigerate: 1 hour

16 oz. cream cheese, softened
1 cup grated sharp cheddar cheese
1/2 cup of Ranch dressing
6 ounces light beer
2 tbs. crushed peanuts

Blend together cheeses, Ranch dressing and beer in food processor. Remove with spatula and shape into ball. Sprinkle crushed peanuts onto ball. Refrigerate. Let sit 15 minutes before serving. Serve with pork rinds or low carb crackers.
Per 2 oz. serving: protein 8g, carbohydrates 5.2g

Cold Peel & Eat Beer Shrimp
Serves 8   I, T, M
Prep Time: 10 minutes, Cook Time: 5 Minutes, Refrigerate: 1 hour

two 12 oz. low carb, lightly-hopped beers
2 lb. large shrimp, uncooked
1 large onion
1 large clove garlic, chopped
1 large slice of lemon
1 tsp. Tabasco sauce
2 tbs. pickling spices
1 bay leaf
coarse or kosher salt to taste
freshly-ground black pepper to taste

Bring the beer to a boil in a large saucepan. Add the onion, garlic, lemon slice, Tabasco, pickling spices, bay leaf, salt and pepper. Boil 5 minutes. Add shrimp, stir and cook for 3-5 minutes, or until they just turn pink. Remove the shrimp from the beer, using a slotted spoon. Cover and refrigerate until ready to serve. Serve with lemon wedges. Peel and eat.
Per serving: protein 28g, carbohydrates 2g

Mushrooms Stuffed With Sausage
Serves 5 I, T, M
Prep Time: 15 minutes, Cook Time: 15 minutes

10 large button mushrooms
1 lb. bulk pork or Italian sausage

1 beaten egg
2 tbs. Parmesan cheese
pinch of salt, pepper

Remove mushroom stems. Finely chop stems. Lightly sauté sausage in a pan and break up the meat as it browns. When slightly browned add the mushroom stems. Continue cooking until sausage is just about done. Drain sausage and mushroom mixture well and cool. In a mixing bowl add egg, sausage and mushroom mixture. Fill mushroom caps and place on baking pan. Sprinkle with cheese. Bake 15 minutes at 375-400°F.
Per serving: protein 24g, carbohydrates 2g

Peach Walnut Brie Torte
Serves 8   I, T, M
Prep Time: 10 minutes, Refrigerate: 1 Hour

14 ounce wheel Brie cheese, well-chilled
2 oz. walnuts, finely chopped
2 tbs. low carb peach preserves or jelly

Carefully cut well-chilled Brie horizontally into halves. Set aside. Spread preserves evenly on cut side of one of the brie halves. Top with other half, cut side down. Press together lightly. Wrap and chill. Serve at room temperature with low carb crackers.
Per serving: protein 8g, carbohydrates 2g

Party Meatballs
Serves 16   I, T, M
Prep Time: 10 minutes, Cook Time: 20 minutes

2 lbs. breakfast pork sausage
1 lb. ground beef
3 eggs
2 tbs. instant minced onion
1/2 lb. sharp cheddar cheese, shredded
1/2tsp. black pepper

Preheat oven to 350°F. Combine all ingredients and pepper to taste in a bowl. Mix thoroughly. Roll into 1-1/2 inch balls or drop by spoonfuls onto non-stick cookie sheet. Bake 18-20 minutes. Makes 50 meatballs.

Two meatballs per serving: protein 15.28g, carbohydrates 1g

Quick & Easy Pate
Serves 8   I, T, M
Prep Time: 10 minutes, Cook Time: 20 minutes

2 lbs. liver sausage
1 clove garlic peeled & sliced
1 tsp. thyme
1/4 tsp. sage
crushed black pepper to taste
salt to taste
1/2 tsp. Dijon mustard
4 oz. heavy cream

Blend all ingredients in a food processor. Spoon mixture into bowl. Chill for 1 hour. Serve with pork rinds or low carb crackers.

4 tsp. per serving: protein 3.7g, carbohydrates 1g

Smoked Fish Pâté
Serves 8 I, T, M
Prep: 15 minutes, Refrigerate: 1 hour

12 oz. whole smoked fish, skinned and de-boned
1/2 lb. cream cheese
2 tbs. mayonnaise type salad dressing
1-1/2 tbs. lemon juice
1/8 tsp. ground black pepper
1 tbs. scallions, minced

Blend fish and next 5 ingredients in a food processor until smooth. Transfer fish mixture to a bowl. Serve immediately or cover and refrigerate. Allow refrigerated pâté to stand at room temperature 15 minutes to soften before serving. Serve with pork rinds or low carb crackers.

2 tbs. per serving: protein 12.5g, carbohydrates 2g

Stuffed Jalapeno Peppers
Serves 6   I, T, M
Prep Time: 10 minutes, Refrigerate: 1 hour

12 pickled jalapeno peppers, whole and drained
8 oz. packaged cream cheese, softened

1/4 tsp. garlic salt
1 tbsp. diced onion
4 tbsp. mayonnaise

Cut each jalapeno pepper in half lengthwise and remove veins and seeds. In a small bowl blend the cream cheese and mayonnaise. Mix in the onion and garlic salt to taste. Stuff the pepper halves with the cheese mixture. Chill 1 hour before serving.
Per serving: protein 7.5g, carbohydrates 2.2g

Dips & Salsas

A great way to enjoy these dips is with pork rinds. With zero carbohydrates to contend with in the pork rinds, you simply have to watch the carbohydrate content of the dips or salsa.

Barney's Clam Dip
Serves 8   I, T, M
Prep Time: 30 minutes

two 8-ounce packages of cream cheese
two 6 ½ oz. cans minced clams with juice
1 tbs. lemon juice
1 tbs. dehydrated onions
1 tsp. Tabasco sauce
2 tbs. Worchestshire sauce
seasoned salt and black pepper to taste.

Put all ingredients in a mixing bowl and let sit for 20-25 minutes until cream cheese is softened. Blend until smooth. Adjust seasonings. Serve with pork rinds or raw vegetables.

Per serving: protein 13.75g, carbohydrates 4.2g

Carne Party Dip
Prep Time: 10 minutes, Cook Time: 40 minutes
Serves 6   T, M

8 oz. cream cheese, softened
1 can beef chili, no beans
1/2 lb. canned chopped green chili peppers
1/2 lb. shredded Mexican blend taco cheese

Preheat oven to 350°F. Spread cream cheese evenly in the bottom of a baking dish. Spread canned chili over cream cheese. Spread diced green chiles over meat. Sprinkle with Mexican blend taco cheese. Bake 40 minutes. Serve with pork rinds.

Per serving: protein 24g, carbohydrates 15.7g

Salsa
Prep Time: 15 minutes, Refrigeration Time: Overnight
Serves 4   I, T, M

2 large tomatoes, chopped
½ cup onion, finely chopped
1/3 cup red bell pepper, seeded and finely chopped
1 Scotch Bonnet pepper, chopped very fine
2 tbs. fresh cilantro, chopped

1 tbs. fresh lime juice
salt to taste

Mix together all ingredients. Cover and refrigerate overnight. Serve with pork rinds.
Per serving: protein <1g, carbohydrates 5.9g

Lite Creamy Spinach Dip
Serves 4   I, T M
Prep Time: 10 minutes, plus refrigeration time

6 tbs. plain yogurt
2 tbs. mayonnaise
1/8 tsp. dried dill weed
1/8 tsp. celery salt
1/2 cup frozen cut leaf spinach, cooked, well drained, cooled slightly
3 tsp. scallions, chopped
2 tsp. red bell pepper (optional), seeded and chopped

Combine first 4 ingredients in a bowl and blend well. Stir in remaining ingredients. Cover and refrigerate several hours to blend flavors. Serve with crisp vegetables or pork rinds.
Per serving: protein 1.6g, carbohydrates 3.85g

Microwave Hot Spinach Dip
Serves 4   I, T, M
Prep Time: 10 minutes, Cook Time: 5 minutes

2 ounces frozen spinach, thawed, squeezed to drain, chopped

2 ounces cream cheese, softened
2 tbs. sour cream
dash of onion powder
1/8 tsp. dried dill weed
1 ounce sliced pimento, drained

Combine all ingredients in a microwave-safe casserole
and mix well. Cover with microwave-safe waxed paper
or plastic wrap. Microwave on HIGH 3-5 minutes or
until hot, stirring twice during cooking. Serve with low
carb crackers and fresh vegetables.
Per serving: protein 2.2g, carbohydrates 2.2g

Grilled Peach and Red Bell Pepper Salsa
Serves 4   T, M
Prep: 15 min, Cook: 10 min

1 tbsp. plus 1 tsp. olive oil
1 tbsp. plus 1 tsp. fresh basil, finely chopped
2 tsp. fresh mint, finely chopped
1 clove garlic, pressed
3 medium peaches, firm but ripe, halved and pitted
1/3 cup bottled roasted red bell peppers, drained and
cut into 1/2 inch pieces
2 tsp. malt vinegar

Pre-heat grill or turn on broiler. Combine first 4
ingredients and salt and pepper to taste in a bowl.
Lightly brush cut side of peaches with half of oil
mixture. Grill or broil peaches about 2 minutes on the
cut side only until golden. Do not allow to burn.
Remove peaches from heat and allow to cool. Chop

peaches and combine with remaining ingredients and oil mixture in a bowl. Season with salt and pepper to taste and toss. Good on fish or chicken.

Per serving: protein 0.4g, carbohydrates 7.7g

Creamy Southwest Dip
Serves 4   I, T, M
Prep Time: 10 minutes

1 ½ cups low-fat cottage cheese
1 jalapeño or serrano pepper, seeded and chopped
1-1/2 tsp. cilantro, minced
1/2 tsp. garlic powder

Combine all ingredients in a bowl. Mix thoroughly and serve with tortilla chips or pork rinds.

Per serving: protein 10.2g, carbohydrates 3.6g

Spinach Artichoke Dip
Serves 4   T, M
Prep Time: 10 minutes, Cook Time: 20 minutes

2 tsp. unsalted butter
2 tbsp. onions, chopped
7 ounces frozen chopped spinach, thawed and drained
9 ounces canned artichoke hearts, drained and chopped
2/3 cup grated Parmesan cheese
1 clove garlic, minced
1/8 tsp. Worcestershire sauce
3/4 tsp. lemon juice

Preheat oven to 350°F. Melt butter in a heavy nonstick skillet over medium high heat. Sauté onion 3-4 minutes until softened. Press out excess moisture from drained spinach. Stir in remaining ingredients and transfer to a baking dish. Bake 20 minutes or until bubbly. Serve with pork rinds.
Per serving: protein 10.4g, carbohydrates 9.4g

Tomatillo & Lime Salsa
Serves 4   I, T, M
Prep Time: 15 minutes, plus refrigeration time.

2 large tomatoes, chopped
2 large tomatillos, husked, washed and chopped fine
1/3 cup red onion, finely chopped
1/3 cup red bell pepper, seeded and finely chopped
2 tbsp. fresh lime juice
2 tsp. lime peel, grated

Mix together all ingredients. Cover and refrigerate overnight.
Per serving: protein 1.7g, carbohydrates 7.8g

Soups

Cold or hot, a cup or bowl of soup can be a satisfying dish and a convenient way to use up leftovers. It's also a rich blend of proteins and carbohydrates. Accompanied by a salad and a beer, soups made during the weekend and portioned to the freezer can be real time savers.

Hot
Cheese and Beer Soup
Serves 6   I, T, M
Prep Time: 10 minutes, Cook Time: 1 hour

6 cups low sodium canned chicken stock
1 cup chopped onion
1 cup chopped celery
1/2 tsp. mustard powder
2 tbsp. vegetable oil
dash Worcestershire sauce
dash Tabasco sauce
ground pepper (to taste)
1 cup extra sharp cheddar cheese
1 lb. smoked polish sausage
1 bottle light beer

Saute celery and onions in 2 tbsp. vegetable oil until onion is soft and translucent. Add broth and boil. Simmer covered 45 minutes to 1 hour. Grate cheese and add to soup. Don't stir for a short while to allow cheese to break up a bit. Add everything else and heat until sausage is hot.
Per serving: protein 30g, carbohydrates 6g

Peanut Soup
Serves 6   I, T, M
Prep Time: 15 minutes, Cook Time: 35 minutes

2 tbs. unsalted butter
2 tbs. onion, minced
1 celery rib, thinly sliced (optional)
2 tbs. all purpose floor
3 cups low-sodium canned chicken stock
1/2 cup creamy peanut butter
2 tbs. lemon juice
2 tbs. roasted peanuts, chopped

Melt butter in a heavy saucepan over low heat. Sauté onion and celery about 5 minutes until softened. Stir in flour until well blended. Stir in chicken stock and simmer over medium heat about 30 minutes. Remove from heat, strain stock and discard solids. Stir in peanut butter, lemon juice and salt to taste into strained broth. Mix thoroughly. Serve hot, garnished with chopped peanuts.
Per serving: protein 8.8g, carbohydrates 8.7g

Pizza Soup
Serves 4   T, M
Prep Time: 10 minutes, Cook Time: 15 minutes

1 tbs. olive oil
1 onion, finely chopped
1/2 cup fresh or canned mushrooms, sliced
1/4 cup green/red bell pepper, thinly sliced

1 cup canned stewed tomatoes, undrained
3 cups canned beef stock
1/2 lb. pepperoni, thinly sliced
1 tsp. Italian herb seasoning
or 2 tsp. fresh basil, chopped fine
1 cup shredded mozzarella cheese

Turn on broiler. Heat oil in a heavy nonstick skillet over medium high heat. Sauté next 3 ingredients 3-5 minutes until softened. Add remaining ingredients, except cheese. Season with salt and pepper to taste. Simmer 5-10 minutes until heated through, stirring occasionally. Transfer soup to ovenproof bowls and sprinkle with cheese. Broil 1-2 minutes until bubbly.
Per serving: protein 21.9g, carbohydrates 9.8g

Roasted Red Pepper Soup
Serves 4   T, M
Prep Time: 20 minutes, Cook Time: 30 minutes

4 medium sized sweet red peppers
1/2 cup green onions, chopped
3/4 tsp. dried thyme
1/4 tsp. salt
1/4 tsp. cracked pepper
2 gloves garlic, minced
1 ¼ cups canned, low-sodium chicken broth
1 tbs. butter
1 tbs. all-purpose flour
1/2 cup half & half
3/4 cup sour cream

Spear pepper with fork and hold over open flame from stove until skin starts to blacken. Place each pepper in paper bag while roasting the others. Rinse whole charred peppers under cold running water while removing blackened skin with knife. Coarsely chop peppers. Place butter in frying pan and add green onions until tender. Add flour and stir until smooth. Add half & half slowly. Cook one minute, stirring constantly. Remove from heat.

Add peppers, thyme, salt, pepper, garlic and ¼ cup chicken broth in a blender and process until smooth. Add remaining broth and run until smooth. Put onion/flour/half & half mixture back under medium heat and add pepper mixture. Cook until bubbly. Mix in ½ cup sour cream and heat thoroughly. Ladle into soup bowls and top off with 1 tsp. of sour cream per bowl.

Per serving: protein 3g, carbohydrates 13.75

Spicy Chicken, Corn, and Tomato Chowder
Serves 4   T, M
Prep Time: 10 minutes, Cook Time: 1 hour.

1 1/2 lbs. chicken, cut up
2 cups water
1/2 medium onion, chopped
1 jalapeno pepper, seeded, chopped
1/2 tsp. taco seasoning
1/2 lb. canned creamed corn
1/2 lb. canned whole tomatoes, preferably Italian, drained and cut up

1/2 tsp. lime or lemon juice

Bring first 4 ingredients to a boil in a large pot over high heat. Simmer 45 minutes. Remove chicken and let cool. Reserve broth and skim fat from top. Remove meat from chicken, discarding skin and bones. Cut meat into bite-size pieces. Knock off 45 minutes cooking time by using 1 pound frozen cut up chicken and 2 cups of canned chicken broth. Combine chicken, chicken broth and remaining ingredients in soup pot. Simmer 15 minutes. Season with salt and pepper to taste.

Per serving: protein 38g, carbohydrates 12g

Salads

Although nothing can beat a simple salad of head lettuce and tomato for time and simplicity, these salads are designed to hold your interest where other low carbohydrate recipes fail. As you'll see, a number of the recipes transcend the mediocrity that can develop in other diets. Virtually all these salads can be considered an accompaniment to the main entrée, or, in the cases of the Sweet & Sour Chicken, Grilled Chicken Salads and the Lobster Salad, the entrée itself.

Grilled Chicken Salad
Serves 4   I, T, M
Prep Time: 10 minutes, Cook: Time 10 minutes, Chill Time.: 1 to 2 hours

2/3 cup mayonnaise
2 tbs. malt vinegar
1 tbs. plus 1 tsp. fresh lemon juice
3/4 tsp. Worcestershire sauce
1 tbs. plus 1 tsp. extra virgin olive oil
1 clove garlic, minced
4 boneless skinless chicken breast halves
1 head of green leaf lettuce

Combine first 6 ingredients and salt and pepper to taste in a bowl. Whisk until smooth. Place in refrigerator. Prepare grill or broiler. Season chicken with salt and pepper to taste. Grill or broil 4-5 minutes per side, until just cooked. Cut diagonally across the grain into 1/4 inch slices. Divide lettuce between individual serving plates. Pour dressing over. Top with sliced chicken breasts.
Per serving: protein 27g, carbohydrates 3.4g

Cucumber Salad
Serves 4   I, T, M
Prep Time: 10 minutes, plus refrigerator time.

2 large cucumbers, peeled, seeded and sliced
1/3 sliced white or yellow onions
1/4 cup white vinegar

1/4 tsp. salt
1/4 tsp. pepper
pinch of fresh or dried dill

Combine all ingredients in a serving bowl. Add freshly ground black pepper to taste. Chill.
Per serving: protein 1.5g, carbohydrates 6.1g

Spinach Salad
Serves 4   I, T, M
Prep Time: 5 minutes

1 lb. spinach leaves, washed and torn into pieces, tough stems discarded
2 cups mushrooms, sliced
1 cup cherry tomatoes, cut in half
1/4 cup Italian dressing
Combine spinach, mushrooms and tomatoes in a salad bowl. Pour dressing over salad and toss.
Per serving: protein 3.4g, carbohydrates 6.9

Sweet and Sour Chicken Salad
Serves 4   T, M
Prep Time: 15 minutes

3/4 lb. boneless skinless chicken breast, cooked and cut into 2 inch cubes
1 cup celery, diagonally sliced
2/3 cup snow peas, trimmed
1/3 cup red bell pepper, seeded and diced

2/3 cup apples, preferably green and tart, unpeeled and diced
2 tbs. malt vinegar
2 tbs. canola oil
1 tbs. Sugar substitute
3/4 tsp. paprika
3/4 tsp. celery seed
salt and pepper, to taste

Combine all salad ingredients. Whisk together the dressing ingredients. Pour the dressing over the salad and serve.

Per serving: protein 20.9g, carbohydrates 10.7g

Cobb Salad
Serves 4   I, T, M
Prep Time: 10 minutes Cook Time: 10 minutes

2 eggs
10 ounces packaged fresh spinach
1 head lettuce, torn into bite size pieces
1/4 cup blue cheese, crumbled
1-1/2 cups cooked turkey or chicken, shredded
1 avocado, sliced
1/2 cup bottled real bacon pieces
1/2 cup lemon herb dressing

Place eggs in a saucepan with water to cover. Bring to a boil over high heat. Reduce heat to medium low and cook 10 minutes. Transfer eggs to a bowl of cold water to cool. Peel and quarter eggs and set aside. Line serving plates with spinach and top with lettuce. Layer

cheese, turkey, avocado, bacon pieces and eggs over top. Drizzle dressing over salad and serve.
Per serving: protein 46.3g, carbohydrates 3g

Wilted Spinach and Bacon Salad
Serves 4   I, T, M
Prep Time: 5 minutes, Cook Time: 10 minutes

4 bacon slices, chopped into small pieces
1 lb. fresh spinach, finely shredded

Heat a heavy nonstick skillet over medium high heat. Cook bacon 4-5 minutes or until almost crisp. Add spinach and salt and pepper to taste. Sauté 3-4 minutes, stirring occasionally until spinach is just wilted. Serve hot.
Per serving: protein 5.3g, carbohydrates 2g

Lobster Salad
Serves 4   I, T, M
Prep Time: 10 minutes

1/2 lb. cooked lobster meat
1/4 cup fresh button mushrooms, sliced
1 small green bell pepper, seeded and sliced
2 tbs. olive oil
1/4 tsp. Italian herb seasoning
4 green leaf lettuce leaves
2 tsp. fresh lemon juice
2 tbs. Parmesan cheese

Combine first 5 ingredients in a bowl. Serve on lettuce drizzled with fresh lemon juice and sprinkle with Parmesan cheese.
Per serving: protein 13.3g, carbohydrates 3g

Entrees
Egg Dishes
Baked Eggs Florentine
Serves 4   I, T, M
Prep Time: 5 minutes, Cook Time: 15 minutes

10 ounces frozen chopped spinach, thawed
1/2 cup half and half
1/4 tsp. grated nutmeg
8 eggs
1 cup Swiss cheese, grated

Preheat oven to 325°F. Squeeze out as much water from the spinach as possible. Spread spinach in bottom of 4 lightly buttered shallow ramekins or individual gratin dishes. Drizzle each with 1 tbs. half and half. Season with nutmeg and salt and pepper to taste. Carefully break 2 eggs into each dish. Drizzle with remaining half and half and sprinkle with cheese. Bake 12-15 minutes, until whites are just set and cheese is melted.
Per serving: protein 22.6g, carbohydrates 5.4g

Denver (Western) Omelet
Serves 2   I, T, M
Prep Time: 10 minutes, Cook Time: 5 minutes

4 eggs
½ cup green peppers
4 mushrooms, thinly sliced
1/2 cup chopped onions
1 oz. slice of boiled ham, chopped
1 slice cheese, your choice
1 tbs. butter

Melt butter in non-stick pan. Add peppers, mushrooms, onions and ham. Cook until onions are soft and translucent. Scramble eggs in a bowl and add to pan. When eggs start to set up, add cheese. Fold over mixture when firm and serve.
Per serving: protein 19g, carbohydrates 8.75g

Deviled Eggs
Serves 4   I, T, M
Prep Time: 5 minutes. Cook Time: 7 minutes

4 eggs
2 tbs. mayonnaise
1 pinch. paprika, garlic powder, black pepper
2 shakes of Tabasco sauce

Boil eggs for 7 minutes. Plunge into cold water for 5 minutes. Peel eggs and slice length-wise. Remove yolks to mixing bowl. Add all other ingredients and puree with fork until smooth. Scope mixture back into eggs and serve. Add chopped herbs such as dill, basil, etc. for variety.

Per serving: protein 6g, carbohydrates < 1g

Egg Foo Yong
Serves 4   I, T, M
Prep Time: 10 minutes, Cook Time 10 minutes

6 eggs
1/2 cup chopped green onions
1/2 tsp. salt
16 oz. can of beans sprouts, drained and rinsed
4 tbs. oil for frying
****

Sauce
1 tbs. cornstarch
1 tsp. sugar substitute
1 chicken bouillon cube
pinch of ground ginger
1 cup of water
2 tbs. soy sauce

Pre-heat oven to 300 to hold cooked patties. In mixing bowl, beat eggs and add green onions, salt and bean sprouts. Mix thoroughly. Drop mixture into frying pan with heated oil, splitting into 4 patties. Fry until golden brown and turn over. Cook through. Drain on paper towels. Place patties on heat resistant plate and put in oven to keep warm.

Combine cornstarch, sugar substitute, bouillon cube and ground ginger into small saucepan. Cook until

mixture thickens, stirring constantly. Serve with patties.
Per serving: protein 14g, carbohydrates 12g

Eggs and Lox
Serves 4   I, T, M
Prep: 5 minutes, Cook Time: 5 minutes

1/4 cup unsalted butter
1-1/3 cups onions, minced
1/2 lb. lox or smoked salmon, chopped
8 eggs, beaten

Melt butter in a heavy nonstick skillet over low heat. Sauté onions 3-4 minutes until very soft but not brown. Stir in lox and cook 1-2 minutes. Add eggs. Turn heat to low and gently stir until eggs are set. Serve immediately.
Per serving: protein 23.5g, carbohydrates 5.8g

Pepper Frittata
Serves 8 I, T, M
Prep Time: 15 minutes, Cook: 20 minutes

1/4 cup olive oil
3 red bell peppers, seeded and cut into 3/4 inch squares
2 green bell peppers, seeded and cut into 3/4 inch squares
1 onion, finely chopped
1 clove garlic, minced
1 jalapeño pepper, seeded and minced
1 tsp. dried basil

1 tsp. malt vinegar
8 eggs, beaten
3/4 cup Provolone cheese, shredded
1/2 cup grated Parmesan cheese

Preheat oven to 350°F. Heat oil in a flameproof casserole or deep oven proof nonstick skillet over medium high heat. Stir in next 7 ingredients and salt to taste. Sauté 8-10 minutes, stirring frequently, until peppers are cooked through. Reduce heat to medium. Stir in vinegar and pepper to taste. Stir provolone cheese into eggs and season with salt and pepper to taste. Pour egg mixture over vegetable mixture, swirling skillet to distribute eggs evenly. Cook 2 minutes. Sprinkle with Parmesan cheese. Transfer to oven and bake about 10 minutes, or until frittata is just set in center. Remove from oven and let stand 15 minutes. Run a knife around edges to loosen frittata from sides of pan. Cut into wedges and serve.

Per serving: protein 13.6g, carbohydrates 12.7g

Salami and Onion Scrambled Egg
Serves 4   I, T, M
Prep Time: 5 minutes, Cook: Time 5 minutes

1 tbsp. unsalted butter
1/2 lb. hard salami, 1/4 inch thick, cut into strips
8 eggs, lightly beaten
1/4 cup chopped onion
Heat oil in a heavy nonstick skillet over medium high heat. Sauté salami strips and chopped onion 3-4

minutes until lightly browned. Add eggs and stir 1-2 minutes, until just set.
Per serving: protein 13g, carbohydrates 1g

Meats
Beef
Beef and Chili Relleno Casserole
Serves 8   I, T, M
Prep Time: 10 minutes, Cook Time: 55 minutes

1 lb. ground beef
1 1/2 cups onion, chopped
1/2 lb. green chilies, cut and seeded
1 1/2 cups shredded cheddar cheese
1 cup half & half
1/4 cup all purpose flour
4 eggs, beaten

Preheat oven to 350°F. Heat a heavy nonstick skillet over medium high heat. Sauté meat and onions 5-7 minutes, stirring frequently until meat is brown and onion is tender. Drain and discard fat. Season with salt and pepper to taste. Place chilies in a 10x6 inch baking dish. Sprinkle with cheese, then top with meat mixture. Combine remaining ingredients in a bowl. Mix thoroughly until smooth. Pour over meat-chili mixture. Bake 40-45 minutes. Let cool before serving.
Per serving: protein 22.7g, carbohydrates 9g

Beef 'n' Beer
Serves 12
Prep Time: 10 minutes, Cook Time: 2.5 hours

4 lb. boneless chuck
1 tsp. seasoned salt & pepper
2 large onions, thinly sliced
6 large carrots sliced thick
8 oz. package mushrooms sliced into chunks
12 oz. light beer
1 tsp. hot mustard

Salt & pepper meat and brown lightly in heavy skillet. Add onions and carrots and brown lightly. Pour in beer. Stir in mustard. Cover tightly and simmer slowly for 2 to 2 ½ hours or until meat is tender. Add mushrooms last 15 minutes.

Per serving: protein 43g, carbohydrates 4.5g

Blue Cheese Burgers
Serves 4   I, T, M
Prep Time: 5 minutes, Cook Time: 10 minutes

1/3 cup blue cheese, crumbled
1 egg
1/4 tsp. onion salt
1 tbs. Worcestershire sauce
1 lb. lean ground beef

Prepare grill or turn on broiler. Combine all ingredients in a bowl and mix thoroughly. Shape into 4 patties.

Grill or broil 4-5 minutes per side or to desired doneness.
Per serving: protein 32.5g, carbohydrates 3.5g

Chateau Briand
Serves 6   I, T, M
Prep Time: 10 minutes, Marinate Time: 1 hour, Cook time: 45 minutes

2 tbsp. lemon juice
2 tbsp. olive oil
1 clove garlic, mashed
2 lbs. beef tenderloin
1 tsp. Beau Monde seasoning
1/2 cup canned low sodium beef stock
2 tbsp. unsalted butter
1 bottle light beer

Combine first 3 ingredients in a bowl. Pour in beer and mix. Place tenderloin in marinade. Marinate 1 hour. Remove from marinade. Discard marinade. Preheat oven to 450°F. Sprinkle steak with Beau Monde seasoning and add pepper to taste. Place tenderloin on a rack in a shallow roasting pan. Discard marinade. Sprinkle with Beau Monde seasoning and pepper to taste. Roast uncovered 45 minutes without basting. Transfer roast to a platter, tent with foil and keep warm. Add beef stock to pan and bring to a boil over medium high heat. Add butter and stir until melted. Season with salt and pepper to taste. Slice meat across the grain and serve with sauce.
Per serving: protein 32.5g, carbohydrates 1g

Enchilada Pie
Serves 12   T, M
Prep Time: 10 minutes, Cook Time: 30 minutes

2 lbs. lean ground beef
1 packet taco seasoning mix
one 14 oz. can enchilada sauce
1 can condensed cream of mushroom soup
1 can condensed cream of chicken soup
6 ounces corn tortillas, cut into quarters
2 cups shredded cheddar cheese
1 onion, diced
1/4 cup picante sauce, or to taste

Preheat oven to 350°F. Combine beef and taco seasoning in a heavy nonstick skillet over medium high heat. Sauté meat 5-10 minutes until browned. Drain well. Combine beef, enchilada sauce and soups in a bowl. Mix thoroughly. Arrange tortilla pieces in the bottom of a 9x11 inch baking dish. Cover with beef mixture and sprinkle with cheese and onion. Bake 30 minutes, or until cheese is bubbly. Serve with picante sauce, if desired. Check Appendix for lower carb tortilla chips.
Per serving: protein 23.1g, carbohydrates 11.7g

Grilled Skirt Steak with Cilantro Jalapeño Salsa
Serves 4   I, T, M
Prep Time: 10 minutes, Cook Time: 10 minutes

1/4 cup fresh flat-leaf parsley or cilantro, minced
2 cloves garlic, minced and mashed to a paste with salt to taste
4 small pickled jalapeño chilies, seeded and minced
1/2 cup plain yogurt
1 lb. skirt steaks, scored crosswise

Prepare barbecue grill. Combine first 4 ingredients and salt and pepper to taste in a bowl. Mix well. Season steak with salt and pepper to taste. Grill steak about 6 inches from hot coals 3-4 minutes per side, or until desired doneness. Transfer to a cutting board and let stand 5 minutes. Cut into thin slices across the grain. Serve with salsa.
Per serving: protein 22.9g, carbohydrates 2.9g

Spicy Beef Stir-Fry
Serves 4   I, T, M
Prep Time: 15 minutes, Cook Time: 10 minutes

2 tbsp. vegetable oil
1 tsp. ground cumin
1 tsp. dried oregano leaves
1 clove garlic, minced
1 red bell pepper, seeded and cut into thin strips
1 medium onion, cut into thin wedges

1 jalapeño pepper, seeded and cut into slivers
1 lb. beef top round steaks, cut into 1/8 inch strips
3 cups romaine lettuce, cut in 1/4 inch slices
1/4 cup cilantro, chopped
1/2 cup bottled tomato salsa

Combine first 4 ingredients in a bowl. Heat half the seasoned oil in a heavy nonstick skillet over medium high heat. Sauté bell pepper, onion and jalapeño pepper 2-3 minutes or until just tender. Remove and reserve. Increase heat to high and heat remaining seasoned oil in same skillet. Stir-fry beef strips 1-2 minutes, in batches if necessary, until just cooked through. Return vegetables to pan and heat through. Serve beef mixture over lettuce. Top with cilantro and salsa.
Per serving: protein 29.7g, carbohydrates 4.4g

Lamb
Grilled Butterflied Leg of Lamb
Serves 10   I, T, M
Prep Time: 5 minutes, Cook Time: 1:40 minutes

5 lbs. boneless leg of lamb, butterflied
1/4 cup olive oil
3 tbsp. dried Greek oregano, crumbled
1 tsp. salt
1 clove garlic

Prepare grill. Brush lamb with oil. Sprinkle with oregano and salt. Make small cuts in the lamb and force in bits or slices of garlic. Grill over medium heat 15-20 minutes per pound, turning occasionally and basting with oil until meat thermometer reads 140°F for medium done meat. Let stand 10 minutes before slicing.

Per serving: protein 48.4g, carbohydrates 0.3g

Lamb Burgers
Serves 4   I, T, M
Prep Time: 10 minutes, Cook Time: 5 minutes

1 lb. ground lamb
1 tbsp. plus 1 tsp. plain nonfat yogurt
1-1/4 tsp. fresh Greek oregano, minced
3/4 tsp. fresh thyme, minced
1 tbsp. plus 1 tsp. lemon juice
2 garlic cloves, finely minced

Prepare an outside grill with an oiled rack set 4 inches above the heat source. On a gas grill, set the heat to medium. Combine the meat with the remaining ingredients. Shape into 4 patties. Grill the burgers, turning once, 8 minutes for medium, or 10 minutes for well done.

Per serving: protein 26.2g, carbohydrates 1.8g

Pork
Pork with Peanut Sauce
Serves 4   I, T, M
Prep Time: 15 minutes, Cook Time: 15 minutes

2 tsp. peanut oil
1 ½ lb. pork tenderloins, cut into 1/4 inch slices, each slice cut in half
1/2 tsp. chili pepper flakes
1/2 tsp. ground ginger or 1 tsp. fresh, shredded
½ cup water
1/4 cup peanut butter
2 tbsp. soy sauce
1/4 cup scallions, sliced

Heat oil in a heavy nonstick skillet over medium high heat. Cook pork, chili pepper and ginger 5-6 minutes, stirring occasionally until pork is cooked throughout. Transfer pork to a mixing bowl and keep warm. Discard cooking oil. Add peanut butter, 1/2 cup water and soy sauce to skillet, stirring until hot, adding more cooking water if needed. Stir in remaining ingredients and peanut sauce into pork. Serve immediately.
Per serving: protein 29.9g, carbohydrates 6.3g

Mustard-Grilled Pork
Serves 4   I, T, M
PrepTime: 40 minutes, Cook Time: 8-10 minutes

2 lbs. boneless pork chops, 3/4 inch thick
1 ½ cup plum tomatoes, diced

2 tbsp. dijon-style mustard
1 tsp. minced garlic
1/4 tsp. cayenne pepper
¼ cup fresh basil, chopped

In a medium bowl combine plum tomatoes, chopped basil and cayenne; set aside. In a small bowl combine mustard and garlic. Rub mustard mixture over all surfaces of chops. Place chops on a kettle-style grill directly over medium-hot coals, close grill hood and grill for 3-4 minutes. Turn chops and grill for 3-4 minutes more or until chops are just done. Serve with tomato mixture.

Per serving: Protein 56g Carbohydrates 4g

Pork Chops Ole
Serves 4   I, T, M
Prep Time: 10 minutes, Marinate Time: 4 hours +, Cook Time: 15 minutes

1/2 cup canned green chilies, chopped
2 tsp. oregano
2 cloves garlic, minced
2 tsp. ground cumin
1/4 cup malt vinegar
4 pork chops, 1-1/2 inch thick
2 tsp. oil

Place first 5 ingredients in a food processor or blender and purée until smooth. Arrange pork in bottom of a non-reactive pan or dish. Pour vinegar mixture over chops, turning to coat. Cover and marinate chops in mixture 4-24 hours in refrigerator. Heat oil in a heavy nonstick skillet over medium high heat. Remove chops from marinade and pat dry. Discard marinade. Sauté chops 7-8 minutes per side, until just cooked throughout.

Per serving: protein 30g, carbohydrates 4.3g

Fish
Broiled Crab Cakes
Serves 6   I, T, M
Prep Time: 10 minutes, Cook Time: 10 minutes

1-1/2 lbs. fresh crabmeat, cartilage and shells removed
2 tbsp. mayonnaise
2 tbsp. Dijon mustard
3 tbsp. minced onion
1 egg
1/8 tsp. hot red pepper sauce

Combine all ingredients and shape into 6 patties. Broil 6 inches from heat source, 3-5 minutes per side, until golden brown. Patties can also be pan-fried. Serve immediately.

Per serving: protein 28g, carbohydrates 3.3g

Broiled Rainbow Trout with Cream
Serves 4   I, T, M
Prep Time: 5 minutes, Cook Time: 15 minutes

four 12-ounce trout, cleaned, with head and tail left on
2 tbsp. oil

3/4 cup heavy cream, hot
1 tsp. dried tarragon, crumbled or 1 tbsp. fresh, chopped
1 tbsp. parsley, chopped

Turn on broiler. Sprinkle inside of fish with salt and pepper to taste. Rub outside with oil. Place fish in a shallow baking pan and broil 5 inches from heat source 3 minutes. Carefully turn and broil another 3 minutes. Combine tarragon and hot cream and pour over fish. Broil another 3-5 minutes, occasionally spooning cream over fish until cooked through. Serve sprinkled with parsley.
Per serving: protein 72g, carbohydrates 1.4g

Broiled Salmon with Tarragon Butter
Serves 4   I, T, M
Prep Time: 5 minutes, Cook Time: 10 minutes

1/4 cup plus 2 tbsp. unsalted butter
3 tbsp. lemon juice 1 tsp. black pepper
four 6-ounce salmon fillets, 1 inch thick
2 tsp. dried tarragon, crumbled or 3 tbsp. fresh, minced

Preheat broiler. Melt butter with lemon juice in a saucepan over low heat. Remove from heat and add pepper. Arrange salmon, skin side down, on broiler proof pan. Brush with half of butter mixture. Season with salt to taste. Broil 5 inches from heat source 8-10 minutes or until fish is no longer pink inside. Stir tarragon into remaining butter mixture and serve over salmon.

Per serving: protein 42g, carbohydrates 1.5g

Cajun Blackened Snapper
Serves 4   I, T, M
Prep Time: 10 minutes, Cook Time: 5 minutes

four 6-ounce skinless red snapper fillets
1 tbsp. plus 1 tsp. blackened spice seasoning blend
1 tbsp. plus 1 tsp. unsalted butter, melted
1/4 cup fresh-squeezed lemon juice

Heat a heavy nonstick skillet over medium high heat 10 minutes, until very hot. Pan is correct temperature if a drop of water evaporates almost immediately when dropped on surface. Sprinkle seasoning over both sides of fish to coat well. Sear fish in hot pan 2-3 minutes, until bottom is dark brown. Turn and cook another 2 minutes. Drizzle 1/2 tsp. butter over each fillet. Serve immediately. Pour on remaining butter and drizzle with lemon juice.
Per serving: protein 42g, carbohydrates 2.1g

Grilled & Dilled Salmon
Serves 4   I, T, M
Prep Time: 5 minutes, Cook Time: 15 minutes

2 tbsp. unsalted butter, melted
1/2 tsp. dill weed
1/4 tsp. onion powder
1 tbsp. lemon juice
1/8 tsp. pepper

1 lb. salmon fillets

Prepare grill. Combine first 5 ingredients in a bowl and set aside. Spread butter mixture over fillets. Place fish on grill over hot coals. Cook about 15 minutes, until fish flakes when tested with a fork.

Per serving: protein 27.7g, carbohydrates .4g

Halibut with Basil
Serves 4   I, T, M
Prep Time: 10 minutes, Marinate Time: 15 minutes, Cook Time: 20 minutes

1/2 cup light beer
1 tsp. dried basil or 2 tbs., fresh, chopped
2 tsp. olive oil
1/2 tsp. pepper
4 cloves garlic, minced
four 6-ounce halibut steaks
8 slices Bermuda onion, separated into rings
1 lemon, thinly sliced

Combine first 5 ingredients in a baking dish. Add fish in a single layer, turning to coat. Place onion and lemon slices over fish. Cover and marinate in refrigerator 15 minutes. Preheat oven to 350°F. Bake fish 15-20 minutes.

Per serving: protein 42g, carbohydrates 3.6g

Salmon Loaf
Serves 4   I, T, M
Prep Time: 10 minutes, Cook Time: 40 minutes

1 lb. canned salmon, drained and picked over
1/4 cup dry breadcrumbs
1 cup mayonnaise
1/2 cup plus 2 tbsp. onion, chopped
1/4 cup celery, chopped
1/4 cup green bell pepper, seeded and chopped
1 egg
1/2 cup sour cream
1/2 cup cucumber, finely chopped
1/2 tsp. dill weed

Preheat oven to 350°F. Combine salmon and breadcrumbs in a bowl. Stir in half the mayonnaise and 1/2 cup of the onion. Add celery, green pepper and egg. Season with salt and pepper to taste. Mix thoroughly. Shape into a loaf and place in a shallow baking dish. Bake 40 minutes. While salmon is baking, combine remaining mayonnaise and onion in a blender or food processor. Add sour cream, cucumber and dill weed. Process until smooth. Serve salmon loaf with sauce. Can also be formed into patties and fried.
Per serving: protein 30g, carbohydrates 8.5g

Shrimp Dijon
Serves 4   I, T, M
Prep Time: 5 minutes, Cook Time: 5 minutes

2 cups heavy cream
2 tbsp. Dijon mustard
2 tbsp. parsley, chopped
1/2 tsp. grated nutmeg
1/2 tsp. lemon juice
2 tbsp. unsalted butter
1 lb. shrimp, peeled and deveined

Combine first 5 ingredients and pepper to taste in a saucepan over medium high heat. Simmer 4-5 minutes, until reduced to about 1 cup. Melt butter in a nonstick skillet over medium high heat. When butter begins to bubble, add shrimp and sauté 3-4 minutes until pink. Do not overcook.
Per serving: protein 28g, carbohydrates 5.1g

Steamed Mussels In Beer
Serves 4   I, T, M
Prep Time: 10 minutes, Cook Time: 15 minutes

40 mussels
24 oz. light beer
1/2 cup onion, finely diced
4 medium crushed garlic cloves
1/2 cup melted unsalted butter

Make sure all of the mussels are clean and alive. Remove beards. Put into a large pot. Add the onion, garlic and beer. Bring to a boil and reduce to medium heat. Continue to cook until all of the shells are open, about 15 minutes. Discard those that do not open. Pour in melted butter.

Ladle out into individual bowls with beer/butter broth.

Per serving: protein, 45g, carbohydrates, 1g

Scallops with Peppers
Serves 4   I, T, M
Prep Time: 10 minutes, Cook Time: 5 minutes

2 tbsp. plus 2 tsp. unsalted butter
1 lb. sea scallops
1 red and green bell peppers, seeded and sliced
1 jalapeño or serrano pepper, minced
3/4 tsp. garlic salt
2 tbsp. plus 2 tsp. lime or lemon juice

Melt butter in a heavy nonstick skillet over medium heat. Add peppers and cook 3 minutes. Add scallops and cook 3-5 minutes. Season with garlic salt and pepper to taste. Add lime or lemon juice and serve immediately.

Per serving: protein 28g, carbohydrates 7.9g

Shrimp with Basil and Hot Chilies
Serves 4   I, T, M
Prep Time: 15 minutes, Cook Time: 5 minutes

1 lb. cooked shrimp, shelled and devined
1 cup fresh basil, chopped
2 cloves garlic, minced
3 red or green chilies (serrano or fresh jalapeño), seeds removed, thinly sliced
4 green onions, chopped, white and green separated
1 tsp. oil
1/4 cup plus 2 tbsp. canned and low-sodium chicken stock
2 tbs. oyster sauce
2 tbsp. soy sauce

Wash and dry the basil; set aside. Heat a wok or heavy skillet over high heat; add the oil and 2 tbsp. stock, the white part of the scallions, the garlic and chilies; cook for 10 seconds. Add the shrimp. Stir-fry 20 seconds. Add the oyster sauce, the soy sauce, remaining stock and the green part of the scallion. Bring to a boil. Stir in the basil. Cook for 20 seconds.

Per serving: protein 28g, carbohydrates 8.1g

Poultry
Beer Can Chicken
Serves 4   I, T, M
Prep Time: 5 minutes, Cook Time: 45 minutes

1 ½ lb. chicken fryer
1 can beer
1 tsp. seasoned salt
1 tsp. Paprika

Open a can of beer. Sprinkle seasoning on chicken. Stick beer can up cavity of chicken. Place chicken and beer on hot grill, standing up. Try different styles of beer for different flavors. Cook 45 minutes or until done. If you can't get the chicken to stand up, place it on grill with open can of beer next to it.
Per serving: protein 42g, carbohydrates 1g

Chicken Parmigiana
Serves 4   T, M
Prep Time: 5 minutes, Cook Time: 25 minutes

1/3 cup dry bread crumbs
2 tbs. grated Parmesan cheese
3/4 tsp. Italian herb seasoning
1/2 tsp. garlic powder
1 lb. boneless skinless chicken breast halves
1 egg, beaten
1 cup tomato sauce
3/4 cup shredded mozzarella cheese

Bob Skilnik

Preheat oven to 375°F. Combine first 4 ingredients in shallow bowl. Dip each chicken breast in beaten egg, then roll in breadcrumb mixture to evenly coat. Place chicken on a Pam-sprayed cookie sheet. Bake 10 minutes. Turn chicken over and bake another 10-12 minutes, or until chicken is thoroughly cooked. Spoon tomato sauce over chicken. Sprinkle cheese over top. Bake 3 minutes or until cheese is melted.

Per serving: protein 36.3g, carbohydrates 10.5

Cream of Mushroom Chicken
Serves 4   I, T, M
Prep Time: 10 minutes, Cook Time: 1 hour

1 tsp. onion powder
1/2 tsp. paprika
1/4 tsp. garlic powder
1/4 tsp. pepper
1 ½ lbs. skinless, boneless chicken breast, cut into pieces
11 ounces condensed cream of mushroom soup
1/3 cup heavy cream
1 small red bell pepper, chopped
1/2 cup scallions, sliced

Preheat oven to 375°F. Combine first 4 ingredients in a bowl. Place chicken in a baking dish and sprinkle with seasoning mixture. Bake 30 minutes. Combine soup and next 3 ingredients in a bowl. Spoon over chicken. Bake 30 minutes more or until chicken is no longer pink and juices run clear. Stir and serve.

Per serving: protein 54.5g, carbohydrates 5.5

Drunken Chicken
Serves 4 I, T, M
Prep Time: 10 minutes, Cook Time: 20 minutes

1 1/2 lb. skinless and boneless chicken breast, cut into large pieces
2 green peppers cut into thin slices
1 red onion cut into thin slices
1 jalapeno pepper diced, with seed
1 minced clove of garlic
1 can Mexican-styled stewed tomatoes
1 tsp. ground chili pepper
1 tsp. ground cumin
2 tbsp. oil
12 oz. light beer
salt & pepper to taste

Heat the oil in a skillet or frying pan. Salt and pepper chicken. Place chicken in the oil and fry chicken on each side until lightly browned, remove the chicken and set aside. In the same oilsaute the onions, green peppers and garlic for about 2-5 minutes. Add the chicken, tomatoes and beer. Bring to boil, reduce the heat and let it simmer until the chicken is done and the beer is almost absorbed.

Per serving: protein: 42g, Carbohydrates 7.2g

Mustard Grilled Turkey Breasts
Serves 4   I, T, M
Prep: 10 minutes, Cook Time: 10 minutes

four 4-ounce turkey breast fillets
2 tbs. Dijon mustard
2 cloves garlic, minced
1/2 tsp. rosemary
1/4 tsp. pepper
1 tbs. olive oil

Preheat grill or broiler. Combine all ingredients, except turkey, in a jar with a tight fitting lid. Shake vigorously. Grill or broil turkey breasts 4 minutes per side. Spread half the mustard mixture over one side of turkey breasts and grill or broil 3 minutes. Turn and coat with remaining mustard mixture. Broil another 3 minutes or until turkey is cooked throughout.

Per serving: protein 27g, carbohydrates 1.2g

Vegetable Dishes
Baked Eggplant
Serves 4   I, T, M
Prep Time: 15 minutes, Cook Time: 1 hour

2 tsp. olive oil
1/2 onion, chopped
1 clove garlic, minced
1/2 lb. crushed tomatoes
1/2 cup dry white wine or vegetable stock
1 tsp. oregano, or 1-1/2 tbs. fresh, chopped

1 lb. eggplant, peeled and cut into 2 inch pieces
1 cup shredded mozzarella cheese
1/4 cup Parmesan cheese

Preheat oven to 400°F. Heat oil in a heavy flameproof casserole dish or cast iron skillet over medium heat. Sauté onion and garlic 3-4 minutes or until onion is tender. Add tomatoes, wine, oregano and salt and pepper to taste. Increase heat to medium high and simmer 15 minutes. Stir in eggplant and half the mozzarella cheese. Bake 35-40 minutes. Remove from oven and top with remaining cheeses. Bake another 3-4 minutes or until cheese is melted.
Per serving: protein 11.3g, carbohydrates 9.5g

Broccoli Cheese Bake
Serves 6   I, T, M
Prep Time: 10 minutes, Cook Time: 30 minutes

1 lb. broccoli, florets and stems
1 tbs. unsalted butter
1/4 cup onion, finely diced
1 tsp. Worcestershire sauce
1 tsp. lemon juice
1-1/2 tsp. Dijon mustard
1/4 lb. sharp cheddar cheese, shredded
1/2 cup mayonnaise

Preheat oven to 350°F. Place broccoli in a steamer basket over boiling water. Cover saucepan and steam 5-6 minutes. Remove steamer basket from saucepan and set aside. Melt butter in a heavy nonstick skillet

over medium heat. Sauté onion 2-3 minutes or until softened. Remove from heat and stir in Worcestershire sauce and mustard. Add broccoli, cheese, mayonnaise and lemon juice and toss to combine. Transfer mixture to a lightly oiled baking dish. Cover tightly and bake 25 minutes. Remove lid and bake 5 more minutes.
Per serving: protein 9.3g, carbohydrates 4.6g

Broccoli and Cheese Pie
Serves 6   I, T, M
Prep Time: 10 minutes, Cook Time: 55 minutes

1 frozen deep 9-inch pie crust, thawed
4 eggs
1/4 cup light cream
1 cup Swiss cheese, grated
2 cups broccoli florets
pinch of salt and black pepper

Preheat oven to 425°F. Bake crust in oven 10 minutes. Remove from oven. Whisk eggs, light cream, and salt and pepper to taste in a mixing bowl until well-blended. Sprinkle broccoli and cheese over pastry crust. Pour in custard. Bake 15 minutes. Lower heat to 350°F and bake another 30 minutes or until custard is set.
Per serving: protein 13.3g, carbohydrates 15.3g

Creamed Turnips
Serves 4   I, T, M
Prep Time: 10 minutes, Cook Time: 10 minutes

2 cups turnips, peeled and shredded
1 tsp. unsalted butter
1/4 cup heavy cream

Place shredded turnips in a heavy saucepan with just enough water to cover. Bring to a boil over high heat. Remove from. Drain turnips. Rinse under cold water and drain again. Return to saucepan over medium heat. Add remaining ingredients and salt and pepper to taste. Stir occasionally until mixture is hot. Do not boil.
Per serving: protein 2.5g, carbohydrates 8g

Fried Green Tomatoes
Serves 6   T, M
Prep Time: 15 minutes Marinate Time: 20 minutes
Cook Time: 10 minutes

2 lbs. green tomatoes, unpeeled, uncored and cut into 1/2 inch slices
4 eggs, lightly beaten
1 1/4 cups cornmeal
3/4 cup water
1/4 cup vegetable oil
1 tbs. plus 1 tsp. vegetable oil
1/4 cup unsalted butter

Layer sliced tomatoes between several thicknesses of paper towels. Set aside 20 minutes or until most of the moisture is absorbed. Meanwhile, combine beaten eggs with next 3 ingredients and salt and pepper to taste in a bowl. Heat oil and butter in a heavy nonstick skillet over medium high heat until bubbly. Dip tomato slices into batter and cook 3-4 minutes per side until golden brown. Serve at once.

Per serving: protein 6.5g, carbohydrates 13.8g

Green Beans with Mushroom Sauce
Serves 4   I, T, M
Prep Time: 2 minutes, Cook Time: 5 minutes

one 15 ½-16 oz. can green beans, drained
one 14-16 oz. can condensed cream of mushroom soup

Mix both ingredients gently into small pot and heat thoroughly.

Per serving: protein 2g, carbohydrates 7.5g

Grilled Zucchini
Serves 4   I, T, M
Prep Time: 5 minutes, Cook Time: 10 minutes

4 small zucchini, sliced lengthwise in half
1/2 cup Italian-style oil & vinegar salad dressing

Prepare grill. Toss zucchini to coat with Italian salad dressing. Place zucchini on grill over medium heat. Season with salt to taste and cook, turning occasionally and brushing with salad dressing, until zucchini are browned and tender.

Per serving: protein 1.0g, carbohydrates 3.5g

Spinach and Roasted Pepper Casserole
Serves 4   I, T, M
Prep Time: 10 minutes, Cook Time: 20 minutes

1 tbs. unsalted butter
1/2 cup fresh button mushrooms, thickly sliced
1 Bermuda onion, thickly sliced
10 ounces frozen spinach, thawed and squeezed dry
1/4 cup bottled roasted red bell peppers, chopped thickly
1/2 tsp. seasoned salt
1/2 tsp. pepper
1/4 cup feta cheese, crumbled

Preheat oven to 350°F. Melt butter in a heavy nonstick skillet over medium high heat. Sauté mushroom and onion 7-8 minutes until softened. Stir in spinach, peppers and seasoned salt. Mix well. Transfer to a casserole dish and sprinkle with feta cheese. Bake 20 minutes or until heated throughout.

Per serving: protein 6.9g, carbohydrates 5g

Desserts

I've never been a "dessert guy," but when I'm offered a piece of cake, I want to eat the whole thing. Same goes with pies, cookies, etc. When it comes to desserts, the word "moderation" has no meaning. I know my limitations (at least some of them!)

As a result, I've tried to keep away from most desserts. When I do freak out for sweets, I stick with the many low carb fruit-flavored gelatins and creamy puddings available in the diet section of any supermarket. These items, especially the gelatins, can be used throughout the three phases of the diet.

In the Appendix is a listing of web sites that can provide you with a plethora of recipes, including recipes for desserts and a good selection of manufactured dessert items on the low carbohydrate retail market today. For those of you with more control than I can command, please turn to the Appendix.

Chapter 10

F.A.Qs

Q. What should I expect during the first few days of the diet?

A. A lot of things, but let's take it step by step. Here's what I experienced the first few days of the diet.

Day 1—Still working off a carbohydrate rich diet, experienced hunger pangs quite often. Began my first day of the diet with a breakfast of 1/4 cup green peppers mixed with 2 scrambled eggs, 1/2 cup fresh strawberries and a cup of coffee with a teaspoon of half & half. On my back because of a knee injury, I soon started fantasizing a complete gastronomical tour of Chicago from Mr. Beef's Italian-style beef sandwiches with sweet and hot peppers, a quick food fantasy in Chinatown, then to Greektown and finally to Pizzeria Duo for a Chicago-style deep dish pizza. A couple of pieces of salami and a few deviled eggs stopped my cravings and kept me going until lunch and dinner.

Kept a two-liter bottle of seltzer water nearby to satisfy the requirement of drinking eight glasses of water a day. Loaded with nervous energy but with the limitations of a bum knee, I managed to consume two bottles of seltzer while laying on my back.

Day 2—Much like Day 1 but the cravings have started to slow down. Keeping up with my water requirements, I'm heading to the bathroom with much frequency.

Day 3—A little constipated in the morning, something I expected with the lower carbohydrate level during the first three days of the diet. With the higher levels of carbohydrates to be consumed during the next three days, I'm not concerned but will make it a point to up my fiber intake. Feeling a little tired and realized I had forgotten to take a multivitamin for the last three days.

Day 4—Still a bit constipated. My calves are feeling a little tired. I start using Morton's Lite Salt to up my potassium levels, something that often occurs with frequent urination. With a higher level of carbohydrates and fiber, I'm eating more green vegetables to end the constipation.

Day 5—Let's just say that the extra fiber I took in yesterday moved me to a level of relief I haven't experienced in the last few days. Still pissing like a Russian racehorse but my legs are feeling better and I'm losing the feeling of tiredness. The junk food cravings have stopped.

Day 6—Feeling the best I've felt in days, even a bit energy-charged. Got on the scale and found that I'd already lost 8 pounds! From all the trips I've made to the bathroom, I know a lot of this is water, but what the heck…it's 8 pounds. Tried a protein shake with fruit for breakfast this morning. Not bad. I've laid in a supply of sliced turkey, cheese, salami and hard-boiled eggs for quick snacks. Ready for the next 25 days at the 35 grams of carbohydrate level. I'm pumped!

Day 7—Took a look in the mirror today and I'm sure my double chin is actually getting smaller. Even my gut, as round as it is, seems to be on the decline.

Ah, my first beers! Wanting to wholeheartedly enjoy the moment, I poured the bottles of beer into a frosty mug and slowly savored them with my dinner. Made sure to drink a glass of water before and after dinner. The tired feeling in my legs is gone and I find myself with more energy than I've had in months.

Q. **I've heard that low carbohydrate diets are high in fat. What about my cholesterol levels?**

A. Popular consensus among low carbohydrate diet advocates is not to worry about daily fat intake. Of course if you're consuming excessive amounts of carbohydrates while also taking in fat, the dietary fat will not be used as fuel. Any fat intake will go straight to your fat cells or to your liver where it will be turned into cholesterol. By limiting daily carbohydrate intake, the dietary fat will instead be used as a source of energy.

For those of you who are not convinced that fat intake doesn't count, you can easily modify the diet to be low carbohydrate and low fat. Substitute a product like Egg Beaters for fresh eggs. Limit or eliminate fatty cuts of meat and switch to chicken and fish dishes. But be careful. Eliminating fat completely from your diet can cause problems with dry skin, hair loss and brittle nails. Cook with, or use in homemade salad dressings, avocado oil, nut oils such as hazelnut or walnut oil, peanut oil, canola olive oil and sesame oil. Don't forget butter, unless you're hung up on fat intake. It's much more preferable than margarine with its hydrogenated oils.

Q. My (neighbor, wife, friend, etc.) says this is a high protein diet with no fiber. "All you eat is meat!"

A. I used to get upset trying to argue the merits of **The Drink Beer, Get Thin Diet** and any other low carbohydrate diet on the market today. Most of the people who talk against the diet have never read one book about the theory of low carbohydrate living. Going through the pages of this book, you can see that the carbohydrate limitations of the early stages of the diet are peeled away as you get closer to your target weight. By the time you reach your target weight, you will have reached a daily carbohydrate intake that gives you an incredible amount of choices.

As for fiber intake, I look back at my daily food and fiber intake before I created this effective diet and find that I'm eating three times more fiber than I ever did. Alfalfa sprouts, apples, asparagus, blackberries, broccoli, cauliflower, leeks, lettuce, mushrooms, strawberries, sweet peppers…the list of fiber rich fruits and vegetables goes on and on.

Eat at least 25 grams of fiber a day, watch your carbohydrate intake, eat the right fats, keep your protein levels up and enjoy your beer. Then watch how quickly the same people who gave you a hard time about **The Drink Beer, Get Thin Diet** start asking you for dieting advice.

Q. I've gotten dizzy or light-headed during the first week of the diet.

A. The same thing happened to me. Another thing to be aware of is tiredness or soreness in your calves and/or possible leg cramps. Be aware that the diet acts as a diuretic, especially during the first week or so. Because you're off to the bathroom so often, it's essential that you continue your minimum daily consumption of at eight glasses of water a day and replace potassium and sodium which is expelled with all that water. I use Morton Lite Salt to combat these symptoms. It is composed of a mixture of salt and potassium chloride. Sprinkle it on your eggs in the morning or on your vegetables and these reactions will quickly disappear. Potassium supplements will also help.

Q. I got carried away last week-end and drank a six-pack of beer and too many pieces of pizza. Now what?

A. Join the crowd. The first few weeks of the diet are the hardest. They were for me. I had already dropped about 15 pounds and was getting a bit cocky when I knocked off a six-pack of light beer during the third weekend of the diet. I had the presence of mind, however, not to overload on carbohydrates and ate and nibbled my way through low carbohydrate food and snacks including peanuts, salami, deviled eggs and steak while I put down the beers. As a result, I only hit a two-day plateau. It could have been worse.

If you blow the diet with too many beers or high carbohydrate foods, don't whine and mope about it. Get the episode out of the way and move on. Don't wait until tomorrow to resume the diet. Get restarted NOW!

If you're still in the Initial Phase, drop back to 20 grams of carbohydrates for three days and then add five grams more of carbohydrates each day to your daily intake until you reach the 35-grams of carbohydrate level. If you falter in the Transitional Phase, go back to the 35 grams of carbohydrate level for three days and then add five more grams daily to your carbohydrate intake until you reach the level you were at when you slipped. If you falter during the Maintenance Phase, drop back to 55 grams of carbohydrates for three days then add five more grams each day until you reach your previous level of daily carbohydrate intake.

Q. I'm following the diet religiously but have reached a plateau. It's been a week now and I haven't lost a pound. What do I do?

A. The first thing to do is to really look back at your eating regime for the last week or so. Sure you haven't cheated somewhere down the line? All too often, a review of your eating patterns will reveal a flaw.

Did you eat out and accept the waiter's smiling face when he assured you your dish was prepared in a low carbohydrate manner? Was that diet soda really sugar-free?

Those crackers you ate or peanuts you snacked on…did you really count them or just "guesstimate" how many you ate?

One of my brothers-in-law was eating half a bagel with breakfast and couldn't figure why he was stuck at the same weight level. Don't be like him. If you don't understand the theory and practicality of **The Drink**

Beer, Get Thin Diet, go back and read the book again. Start counting your daily carbohydrate level. And please, don't try to fool yourself.

O.K. Let's say you have followed the diet carefully but have stopped losing weight. Have you lost any inches during your plateau? Sometimes your muscle and fat mass is rearranging itself. Be patient. I hit my first long plateau around week six. For almost two weeks I experienced no weight loss. Amazingly, however, I dropped a pants size while trying to figure out what I was doing wrong. Remember, although we all look at a weight reduction program as just that, you will also experience a reduction of body fat. Both features of this diet compliment each other. Relax, have a beer and a snack and go with the flow.

Are you drinking enough water? Cutting back on your water intake can slow down your weight loss. I don't know why but I seem to drink less water on my days off from work and have to consciously work at drinking the minimum of eight glasses of water a day.

If nothing seems to be working, cut back on the carbohydrates for a few days. This might kick-start the resumption of weight loss. If this works, add back carbohydrates daily at five grams increments until you've reached your old level of daily carbohydrate intake.

Q. What about snacks? I feel like I'm cheating when I eat some of the foods listed in the snack section of the recipe chapter.

A. Smart snacking is an important part of the diet. It's also a part of the diet than can cause weight loss plateaus if handled carelessly. Snacking three times a day helps keep your energy level up and your hunger cravings down. However, like the limitation of only two beers a day during the Initial and Transitional Phases, people who have followed this diet admit that they often tried to push the carbohydrate envelope with snacks, especially during the weekends.

I know it might sound silly, but if a serving of roasted peanuts is considered 40 peanuts, don't grab a handful and figure that's a serving. Count the peanuts. If the jar of cheese spread says a serving is two tablespoons, don't just start dipping. Measure out the serving. Don't try to slip in an extra beer or two while you're snacking either.

During the Initial and Transitional Phases of the diet, smart snacking can help you make the diet or break the diet. If you find yourself wavering while snacking, limit your snack times to only once or twice a day rather than three times daily. Use the carbohydrates and protein you saved from not snacking to bolster your intake for the three daily entrees.

Look. This is an unbelievable diet that allows you to do things you could never dream of with a low calorie diet. Beer, peanuts, Slim Jims, big steaks…it's all there for you to enjoy. But as I mentioned in the beginning of the book, moderation is the key.

Q. I really miss bread with my breakfast.

A. A common remark during any lower carbohydrate diet. There are, however, a number of brands of bread on the market that are under 10 grams of carbohydrates per slice, especially after you take the fiber content of the bread into consideration. Try a half-slice or even a slice with some butter and a teaspoon of low carbohydrate preserves. As you progress through the diet and your daily carbohydrate intake increases, this becomes less of an issue.

There are also a number of very low carbohydrate flour replacements on the market that can be used to make muffins, pancakes and breads. No one will confuse these items to taste like something from Mom's kitchen. However, they tend to slow down or stop these cravings for high carbohydrate bread and starch items. A list of companies and web sites selling these products is included in the Appendix.

Q. You can eat all the eggs you want, all the marbled beef you want and can slather butter on your vegetables. However, I'm uncomfortable with the idea of taking in so much fat.

A. Then don't. Although some daily fat intake is necessary, you can control the amount of fat you take in by substituting items, such as Molly McButter for real butter, Egg Beaters or a similar product for eggs and poultry, fish and tofu for beef and pork. I try to maintain a lower level of fat intake but do indulge on occasion, especially on weekends.

Q. Is this a fad diet?

A. Absolutely not! What happens on a low calorie diet? You limit your choice of foods until you lose your desired amount of weight. Slowly you add more foods to your diet until you notice some weight gain…then you cut back again.

What happens when you embark on a low carbohydrate diet? You limit your choice of foods until you lose your desired amount of weight. Slowly you add more foods to your diet until you notice some weight gain…then you cut back again.

Both types of diets share the philosophy of restriction and moderation. Both types of diets strive to achieve the same results. Why should **The Drink Beer, Get Thin Diet** be considered a fad diet? This is a lifetime diet, my lifetime diet, with an emphasis on modification of my old and destructive lifestyle, a diet with quick results and an eating and drinking philosophy that is far more fun than a low calorie diet. It is not a fad diet.

Q. I've looked through all the carb, protein and beer lists and understand the basic philosophy of the diet. Can you show some typical menus for the different phases of the diet?

A. Good question. Here are some examples to give you an idea of how to put the diet together. As you look at the examples, notice the three snacks allowed per day. As you get a better feel for the diet and your daily food needs, you can start skipping or limiting your snacks to allow more carbohydrates during your three daily entrees. You can also limit or even eliminate your beer allowance during those days when (and if) overwhelming hunger cravings take over in order to add additional carbohydrates to the three daily entrees. The choice is yours.

<u>Initial Phase at 20 Carbohydrates, Days 1-3</u>
Breakfast

1/4 cup green peppers
2 eggs scrambled. Mix with peppers
1 pat butter
1/2 cut fresh strawberries
tea, coffee with cream and artificial sugar, if desired

Snack
1/2 cup cottage cheese
1 oz. sliced turkey breast
Lunch
5 Peel & Eat Beer Shrimp *
side salad (head lettuce, cucumber slices, onion, etc.)
1 tbsp. oil & vinegar dressing
diet soda, tea, coffee with cream and artificial sugar, if
desired
Snack
1 deviled egg*
Dinner
4 oz. salmon steak
1 cup steamed broccoli
1 serving cucumber salad *
diet soda, tea, coffee with cream and artificial sugar, if
desired
Snack
1 oz. sliced roast beef
dab of mustard
Total Protein: 90g Total Carbohydrates: 20g
* Recipes included

Initial Phase at 35 Carbohydrates Daily

Breakfast
1 cup puffed wheat
1/2 cup cantaloupe
1/2 cup skim milk
tea, coffee with cream and artificial sugar, if desired

Snack

1 oz. pastrami

1 dill pickle spear

Lunch

4 oz. hamburger patty

1/2 cup brussel sprouts

1 side salad (head lettuce, cucumber slices, onion, etc.)

diet soda, tea, coffee with cream and artificial sugar

Snack

2 tbsp. hummus

small bag of pork skins

Dinner

1 serving Chateau Briand *

1 side salad with bottled blue cheese dressing

2 light beers or 1 equivalent carbohydrate regular beer

1 serving low carb gelatin dessert with ¼ cup blueberries

Snack

1 oz. slice cheese

1 lettuce leaf

40 peanuts

Total Protein: 85g Total Carbohydrates: 35g

* Recipes included

Transitional Phase at 55 Carbohydrates Daily

Breakfast

1 protein shake with ½ cup strawberries

1 low carb bread, toasted, with butter

tea, coffee with cream and artificial sugar, if desired

Snack
1 Slim Jim
1 oz. slice cheese
Lunch
1 boneless, skinless chicken breast
1 cup green beans
1 side salad
1 small apple
diet soda, tea, coffee with cream and artificial sugar, if desired
Snack
1 hard-boiled egg
1 small bag of pork rinds
Dinner
Broiled Crab Cakes *
Broccoli Cheese Bake *
1 side salad
1 tbsp. bottled ranch dressing
1/2 slice low carb bread
1 pat butter
2 light beers or 1 equivalent carbohydrate regular beer
Snack
2 tbsp. cheddar cheese spread
1 slice Wasa Fiber Rye

Total Protein: 100g Total Carbohydrates: 53g
* Recipes included

Maintenance Phase at 100 Carbohydrates Daily

Breakfast
1 slice French toast made with low carb bread
2 strips bacon
1 tbsp. low carb fruit spread
1 cup milk
1 cup tea, coffee
Snack
1 oz. slice salami
1 hard-boiled egg
1 celery stick
1/4 cup sunflower seeds
diet soda, tea, coffee with cream and artificial sugar, if desired
Lunch
1 serving lamb burger *
1 slice low carb bread
1 side salad
1 tbsp. bottled cream of garlic dressing
diet soda, tea, coffee with cream and artificial sugar
Snack
2 tbsp. cream cheese
1 sesame Ry Crisp
Dinner
2 bratwurst
1 cup sauerkraut
1 small potato
2 light or regular beers
1 small apple

Snack
1 oz. slice cheese
1 original Ry Crisp
Total Protein: 88g Total Carbohydrates: 85g w/light beer, 99g w/regular beer
* Recipes included

Bob Skilnik

Appendix

The idea of using carbohydrate restriction in order to lose weight is not new. Various interpretations of low carbohydrate diets have been around since the 1700s. Now with the wide reaching influence of the Internet and a healthy dose of American capitalism, an entire new industry of low carbohydrate products has sprung up in the last few years. Some of these products can be found at your local health food stores, drug stores and the pharmacy sections of supermarkets. Using the Internet, however, one can surf through a much larger and price competitive market.

Of course, along with new products to accommodate the low carb dieter, is a plethora of diet books and supplemental aids that can enhance the dieter's objectives. Doing a search on the Amazon.com web site for "diets" or "dieting," for instance, pulls up over 2500 books on these subjects. Many of the books follow the low calorie philosophy but there are also scores of books and reading supplements for anyone interested in a low carbohydrate approach to weight loss.

The following is just a few of the URLs and addresses for anyone who wants to delve deeper into a better understanding of the numerous diet aids, books and even low carbohydrate support groups that can help you reach the goal of a slimmer, trimmer, healthier and happier you.

Low Carbohydrate Themed Web Sites
The Drink Beer, Get Thin Diet Web Site
URL: http://DrinkBeerGetThinDiet.com

Check our site for updates to carbohydrate counts for both regular and low carb brews. Also contains links to recommended sites.

Aktins & Low Carb Friends Diet Support
URL: http://www.atkinsfriends.com/

"You have found your one site source for lowcarb products, support and motivation! Our marketplace is now open for your lowcarb product needs. Also in our pages, you will find a lowcarb classified section, hundreds of recipes and personal success stories in the faces section, a weight tracker, and daily interaction on our bulletin boards and chat rooms. Several other resources are at your fingertips, so sit back, learn, play and enjoy!" Need I say more?

CARBsmart
URL: http://store.yahoo.com/carbsmart/index.html

Don't pay full-price for your favorite low carb and sugar free items. 10% off suggested retail prices everyday!

ExpertFoods.com
URL: http://www.ExpertFoods.com/

Expert Foods develops and manufactures fine food products for special diets, including low carb. Gives nutritional information for all products. Frozen desserts, cheesecakes, mousse and more. Offers "...special value packages—they could save you $$$$!"

The Low Carb Connoisseur
URL: http://www.low carb.com

A commercial low carb product site. List daily sale and featured items. Sells hundreds of low-carb and sugar free products. Has a search capability. This site beats many of the prices at my local health store including shipping and handling costs. For those of you without web capability, contact them at:

Low Carb Connoisseur,
A Division of The Connoisseur.CC, Ltd.
1520 East Greenville Street Anderson
South Carolina 29621
Telephone numbers: (864) 224-0296 or (888) 339-2477

LowCarb Outfitters
URL: http://www.lowcarboutfitters.com/

Describes itself as selling "The best gear for the low carb journey!" Whatever diet you're on...Atkins,

Protein Power, Carbohydrate Addict's, Sugar Busters…they cover it including bread, chocolate, bread, snacks and tortillas!

netrition.com
URL: http://www4.netrition.com/

A lot of innovative low carb foods here such as pizza kits, pasta, chips, cereals and protein bars. Also offers a newsletter and a health news section.

<u>Additional Web Sites For Low Carb Books</u>
www.amazon.com
http://www.bn.com/

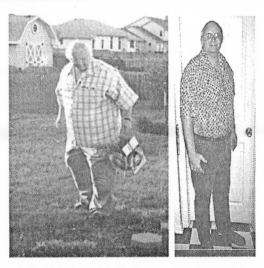

**The author at 305 pounds   Melting away to
230 pounds**

About the Author

Bob Skilnik is a Chicagoland freelance writer and author who has written for <u>The Chicago Tribune</u>, <u>The Collector Magazine</u>, the American Breweriana Association's <u>Journal</u> and the National Association [of] Breweriana Advertising's <u>Breweriana Collector.</u> As a certified brewer, a 1991 graduate of the Chicago-based Siebel Institute of Technology, the oldest brewing school in the United States, he is well versed on the subjects of beer, brewery history and breweriana.

He is a 1991 graduate of the Chicago-based Siebel Institute of Technology, the oldest brewing school in the United States, with a degree in Brewing Technology and has studied beer and brewing with brewers from Miller, Coors, Heineken and numerous micro and regional breweries throughout the United States.

His interests in beer and brewing were cultivated while serving as a German translator in Western Germany for the United States Army. His interest in food was heightened as the owner of a small deli in Chicago.

Skilnik is a former staff writer (now the Associate Editor) for the American Breweriana Association's <u>Journal</u>, the Society of Midland Authors, a contributor to the Smithsonian Institution Traveling Exhibition Service and a member of the Culinary Historians of Chicago. He has appeared in the Chicagoland area on Media One's television program, *The Buzz*, *The Steve*

Edwards Show on Chicago's Public Radio station, WBEZ and the WOR *Morning Show with Ed Walsh* in New York City. He is a frequent lecturer on beer and brewery history.

Skilnik is currently working on contributions to *Alcohol and Temperance in Modern History: An International Encyclopedia*, edited by Huron University College, University of Western Ontario, London, Ontario, Canada. This two part, 500,00-word work will be published by ABC-Clio and available in the Fall of 2003. A pictorial guide of Chicago's old saloon and brewing industries will be available in the spring of 2004. He is also a featured columnist for The Tap, a monthly journal of Chicagoland saloon and tavern culture.

His first book, *The History of Beer and Brewing in Chicago, 1833-1978* was published in 1999 and will soon be available in a second printing. The book was awarded the Quill & Tankard Award by the North American Beer Writers Guild (NABWG) as *"Best Beer Book"* of 1999. The follow up to this work, *The History of Beer and Brewing in Chicago, Volume II,* is now available at the author's website at www.chicagolandbeerhistory.com, www.amazon.com, Infinity Publishing, www.BuyBooksontheWeb.com, local book stores and numerous beer-oriented web sites.